Balance in Healthcare

Authored by

James David Adams

School of Pharmacy University of Southern California
USA

Balance in Healthcare

Author: James David Adams

ISBN (Online): 978-981-4998-96-3

ISBN (Print): 978-981-4998-97-0

ISBN (Paperback): 978-981-4998-98-7

©2021, Bentham Books imprint.

Published by Bentham Science Publishers Pte. Ltd. Singapore. All Rights Reserved.

need for a court order if at any point you breach any terms of this License Agreement. In no event will any delay or failure by Bentham Science Publishers in enforcing your compliance with this License Agreement constitute a waiver of any of its rights.

3. You acknowledge that you have read this License Agreement, and agree to be bound by its terms and conditions. To the extent that any other terms and conditions presented on any website of Bentham Science Publishers conflict with, or are inconsistent with, the terms and conditions set out in this License Agreement, you acknowledge that the terms and conditions set out in this License Agreement shall prevail.

Bentham Science Publishers Pte. Ltd.
80 Robinson Road #02-00
Singapore 068898
Singapore
Email: subscriptions@benthamscience.net

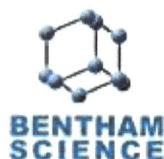

BENTHAM SCIENCE

CONTENTS

PREFACE

Due to the importance of oxygen to conserve and maintain the life of organisms on earth, it is imperative to be conscious of the need for knowledge about this element, its physical, chemical and physicochemical properties, metabolism, and everything related to its behavior and its relationship with living organisms in different ecosystems and environments. Similarly, it is vital to know the causes and serious consequences caused by the incorrect management of natural resources on the levels and quality of this element in the biosphere.

This book presents and analyses evidence of the high enzymatic reactivity of reactive oxygen species, their production sources, chemical formation mechanisms, enzymatic oxidation, reaction centers, mechanisms involved in oxidation-reduction reactions, cell respiration chemistry, enzymatic kinetics, electron transport chain mitochondrial and chloroplast, oxidation-reduction potential, reaction constants, reaction velocity and reaction mechanisms involved, cellular cytotoxicity, antioxidant defense mechanisms in plants and animals, the response of plants to conditions of environmental stress, xenobiotics, heavy metals, paraquat, the thermodynamics inherent to oxygen metabolism. Chapter 5 presents evidence and analyzes the action of flavonoids as promoters of reactive oxygen species. It is written as a paradoxical example of the high reactive affinity of reactive oxygen species for enzymes since during the whole metabolic process that presents flavonoids as trapping agents of reactive oxygen species or oxidants, in the end, and due to this high affinity and reaction rates, they become promoting agents of the same reactive oxygen species.

Dioxide O_2 is not stored in the body. However ambient air (or water) if it is the immediate reservoir of dioxide. The ability to extract oxygen from the environment and carry it to each cell in complex multicellular organisms through just-in-time metabolism was one of the main developments of organisms during evolution. In human cells, there is an increase in reactive oxygen species under conditions of low levels of available oxygen-hypoxia.

The unfortunate experience in which we human beings currently live has alerted all of humanity to the need to take care of nature and the need to have an environment that is as unpolluted as possible since there is sufficient scientific evidence to show the decrease in oxygen levels in the terrestrial and aquatic environments and the devastating effects this has on the survival of organisms. Therefore, there is a need to form citizen conscience about the care of nature and the presence of this essential element for life on earth.

CONFLICT OF INTEREST

The author declares no conflict of interest, financial or otherwise.

ACKNOWLEDGEMENTS

Declared none.

CONSENT FOR PUBLICATION

Not applicable.

James David Adams
School of Pharmacy University of Southern California
USA

CHAPTER 1

Balance and Lifestyle

Abstract: The world is facing a crisis of overpopulation that is confounded by the toxic lifestyles that people choose. The healthcare community must treat the diseases these toxic lifestyles cause, such as heart disease, type 2 diabetes, arthritis, and cancer. Living in balance can prevent and cure these diseases. The public should know more about balance and how to keep the body healthy.

Keywords: Arthritis, Balance, Cancer, Exercise, Heart Disease, Stress, Toxic Lifestyle, Type 2 Diabetes.

1. INTRODUCTION

Balance is a traditional concept that is central to healthcare. Living in balance involves staying thin and strong, being of service to others, having loving relationships with family members, being kind and respectful to other people, and being spiritual [1, 2]. Traditional healers teach that when the body is in balance, it heals itself. It is easy for a doctor to decide if a patient is in balance. The blood pressure, blood glucose, and blood cholesterol are normal.

The modern world is centered around the need to make money. Education focuses on helping people learn how to have lucrative careers. Many people assume they must be aggressive to succeed in their careers. This may add to the stress. Stress is responsible for decreasing balance.

Diet is critical to balance [1, 2]. Many people in the modern world eat diets that emphasize meat and processed foods. Fruit, vegetables, and traditional foods are being ignored. The body needs a balanced diet to keep the guts and the immune system healthy since the immune system has a large component in and near the guts. Insoluble fibers from fruits and vegetables are necessary for gut health and for the health of the immune system.

Toxic lifestyles have become normal in the modern world that leads to obesity [3, 4]. Toxic lifestyles can include alcohol abuse, drug abuse, sexual abuse, obesity, smoking, lack of exercise and other possibilities. In some parts of the world, obesity is a sign of wealth and success, whereas being thin is a sign of poverty. Regular daily exercise is considered nonessential. Exercise is critical to health because muscles need exercise in order to make myokines that maintain the health of the heart, brain, kidneys and other organs. Obesity has become normal in the modern world. Visceral adipocytes secrete inflammatory proteins called adipokines that cause heart disease, type 2 diabetes, osteoarthritis, and promote cancer.

2. LIFESTYLE AND LONGEVITY

The Framingham studies and several other studies have shown the effects of toxic lifestyles on health and longevity [5, 6]. These are studies of several thousand people followed over many years.

1. Smoking, high blood cholesterol, high blood pressure and obesity increase heart disease and decrease life expectancy.
2. Smoking cessation can increase life expectancy.
3. Exercise and elevated HDL levels decrease the risk of heart disease and increase life expectancy.
4. High blood pressure increases the risk of stroke. An enlarged left ventricle, as seen in congestive heart failure, increases the risk of stroke. These factors decrease life expectancy.
5. Never smoking, eating a healthy diet, vigorous daily exercise, maintaining low body weight, and limiting alcohol consumption increase longevity and decrease the risk of developing heart disease, type 2 diabetes, and cancer.
6. 90% of diabetes, 80% of heart disease, 70% of mortality from heart disease, and 50% of mortality from cancer have been attributed to living with toxic lifestyles [6].
7. Processed foods, especially processed meats, increase the risk of developing cancer, according to the World Health Organization.
8. Red meat consumption greatly increases the risk of several intestinal cancers [7].
9. Alcohol consumption increases hypertension [8]. Women have a lower risk of developing alcohol induced hypertension than men. Black people have a higher risk of developing alcohol induced hypertension than whites and Asians. Alcohol consumption damages the guts and can dose dependently increase the risk of cancer [6].

The addition of any aspect of a toxic lifestyle decreases life span and increases the risk of developing heart disease, type 2 diabetes and cancer. These toxic lifestyle aspects include smoking, eating an unhealthy diet, avoiding exercise, obesity and drinking more than 2 alcoholic drinks daily [6]. These toxic aspects are additive in terms of decreasing longevity and increasing disease.

3. HEALTHY DIET

A healthy diet, as defined in the studies discussed here, is described by the alternate healthy eating index [8]. The current recommendations are to eat vegetables, fruit, nuts, soy protein, more white meat than red meat, cereal grain, more polyunsaturated fats than unsaturated fats, multivitamins, and no more than 2 alcoholic drinks daily. Eating a healthy diet is associated with less disease [9].

However, eating too much of a healthy diet can cause obesity. Obesity decreases longevity and increases the risk of type 2 diabetes, heart disease, arthritis and cancer [6]. On the other hand, being too thin also decreases longevity by about 20 – 25 years [6]. Anorexia causes hypoglyccmia, damages the heart and is associated with depression, bipolar disorder, and suicide [10].

For many people, weight loss involves eating less and exercising more [1, 4]. Weight control should become a lifestyle change and should be incorporated into normal life. Dieting without exercise tends to cause loss of muscle tissue. Fad diets are used by many people, usually with limited success. One such diet is the ketogenic diet, which emphasizes eating fat and protein while eliminating carbohydrates. This diet may be useful in the treatment of cancer [11]. However, fibroblast growth factor levels increase during a keto diet [12], which stimulates cell growth, perhaps even cancer growth.

The modern diet is partly the result of wartime rations from World War 2. Some types of processed meat, processed cheese and nonwhole grain flour were promoted for wartime use. Cigarettes were also given in rations to soldiers. Now, these wartime foods are being weaponized against the population as a whole and are greatly decreasing general health. High fructose corn syrup and other flavor enhancers are being added to foods to increase sales. Fat contents of foods are kept high to increase sales. High sugar and high-fat contents cause the release of endorphins and enkephalins in the brain resulting in food addiction [4]. In addition, endocannabinoids are released in the body after high fat and high sugar meals resulting in pleasure and increased appetite [4]. People are choosing to eat more food than is needed for optimal health, resulting in obesity.

The modern diet contains obesogens, which are compounds that stimulate appetite. Many of these compounds stimulate sterol regulatory element binding protein (SREBP). Stimulation of SREBP induces several lipogenic genes responsible for the accumulation of fat and stimulation of appetite. Examples of obesogens include alcohol, phthalates from plastics and bisphenol A from packaging materials [1, 4].

4. SMOKING

Smoking tobacco, *Nicotiana tabacum*, increases the risk of lung, throat, mouth and other cancers [13]. It also increases lung damage such as emphysema and is a leading cause of heart disease [14]. Tobacco contains nicotine that is highly addictive [15]. This makes smoking cessation very difficult.

Nicotine damages arteries and the heart by interacting with non-neuronal nicotinic acetylcholine receptors [16]. The stimulation of these receptors by nicotine results in oxygen radical generation and damage to endothelial cells. Nicotine decreases endothelial progenitor cells that help regenerate damaged arteries [17]. Nicotine damages endothelial cells increases blood triglycerides and decreases HDL [18]. Nicotine upregulates early growth response factor-1 that increases vascular smooth muscle cell proliferation and intimal damage. Nicotine upregulates inflammatory tumor necrosis factor (TNFα), interleukin-2 (IL-2), monocyte chemoattractant protein-1 (MCP-1), intercellular adhesion molecule -1 (ICAM-1), and growth factor receptors for platelet-derived growth factor (PDGF), transforming growth factor (TGFβ) and basic fibroblast growth factor (bFGF). These factors result in more damage to arteries and the heart. Lipid soluble factors in smoke upregulate endothelin receptors and thromboxane A2 receptors that are involved in increased blood pressure and clotting in the arteries [19]. This is why smoking is a major cause of heart disease.

Many species of *Nicotiana* plants are native to South, Central and North America. American Indians have cultivated and used these plants in sacred ceremonies for thousands of years [20]. The sacred ceremony includes the right of passage and other sacred uses. A tea of *Nicotiana* plants has also been used to decrease appetite. When Europeans came to the Americas, they did not learn the sacred uses of *Nicotiana* plants. Instead, they learned to smoke Nicotiana plants socially. Europeans did not learn to respect tobacco.

5. EXERCISE

Human beings have existed for about 500,000 years. During most of this time, we were hunters and gatherers. Running and other strenuous physical exertions are required in order to survive as a hunter gatherer. This has influenced our genetic makeup such that our genes are adapted to running and other strenuous physical activities. For this reason, human beings need physical activity in order to be healthy.

Physical activity is safer and cheaper than drug therapy for healthcare. Physical activity has ameliorative effects on at least 40 diseases, including diabetes mellitus, cancer, cardiovascular disease, obesity, depression, Alzheimer's disease, osteoporosis, and arthritis [21]. In fact, it has been claimed that the best treatment for depression and anxiety is physical activity [22]. Inadequate physical activity causes 9% of premature mortality in the world, or 5.3 million deaths [21]. Smoking causes 5.1 million deaths. At least 80% of American adults do not get adequate physical activity [21].

The health of the vasculature depends on physical activity [21]. Physical activity improves high-density lipoprotein cholesterol, reduces body mass index, improves insulin sensitivity, and reduces blood pressure. Vascular endothelial function and nitric oxide bioavailability increase. Endurance exercise can increase the size of the heart, athletic heart syndrome. This is required for regular endurance exercise and is a sign of good health.

In a study of 82,465 people over 10 years, the weekly exercise of about 75 min increased life expectancy by 1.8 years [23]. Increasing exercise to 450 min per week increased life expectancy by 4.5 years. Exercise was found to be beneficial for life expectancy, even in obese people. It is critical that exercise must be moderate and enjoyable. People should look forward to daily exercise and not seek excuses to avoid exercise.

Does running cause arthritis? There is a major concern in our society that running damages the knees and causes arthritis. In fact, running slows down the progression of arthritis [24 - 30]. All of the evidence from clinical trials shows that running slows down the progression or prevents arthritis. The Framingham and similar studies have all shown that running and other forms of exercise prevent arthritis or slow down the progression of arthritis [5, 21, 23]. Common sense implies that hunters and gatherers who ran daily could not have survived if they were afflicted with arthritis.

Of course, exercise can cause injuries. Excessive use injuries can result from running and other forms of exercise. These injuries usually involve damage to the ligaments, tendons and bones such as plantar fasciitis, shin splints and anterior cruciate ligament injuries.

Another common misconception is that exercise causes myalgic encephalomyelitis/chronic fatigue syndrome. This disease is characterized by excessive, constant fatigue that does not improve with rest and worsens with exertion. The cause of this disease is not known.

Lack of exercise causes muscle loss and fat accumulation. On the other hand, the exercise burns fat and helps build muscle. Trained muscle is required for insulin clearance and healthy glucose tolerance [31]. About 15% of blood insulin is cleared by muscle. Loss of muscle causes blood insulin to increase, resulting in insulin resistance, also known as type 2 diabetes.

Why is muscle important? Muscle secretes myokines that help maintain the health of the heart, kidneys, brain and other organs (Table **1**). Adiponectin is released by muscle and increases glucose transporter 4, glucose uptake and fatty acid oxidation by muscle and other organs [32]. Interleukins are myokines secreted by exercised muscle, including IL6, IL-10, IL-1 receptor antagonists. IL-6 stimulates stem cell production, stimulates glucose production, increases muscle energy [33]. IL-15 decreases fat accumulation [34]. Brain-derived neurotrophic factor (BDNF) is released by muscle in exercise and stimulates fat oxidation [35]. BDNF is released by the brain during exercise and stimulates neurogenesis in the brain [36]

Table 1. Effects of exercise on the body.

Protein Factor	Receptor	Pharmacology
Adiponectin	AdipoR1	Increases glucose uptake, fatty acid oxidation
IL-6	IL6R	Stimulates stem cells and glucose oxidation
IL-15	IL15R	Decreases fat accumulation
BDNF	TrkB, LNGFR	Fat oxidation, brain neurogenesis
Myonectin	Unknown	Fatty acid uptake by liver and fat cells
Decorin	EGFR, TLR2, TLR4	Muscle hypertrophy
Irisin	Integrin $\alpha V/\beta 5$	Brown fat production
Osteonectin	Unknown	Bone mineralization
Leukemia Inhibitory Factor	LIFR	Muscle growth and regeneration
FGF21	FGF21 receptor	Tissue repair

Myonectin production is induced by exercise, stimulates fatty acid oxidation and uptake by fat and liver cells [37]. Decorin is released during exercise and increases muscle hypertrophy [38]. Irisin is released during exercise, decreases white fat development and increases brown fat production [39]. Osteonectin is released during exercise and stimulates bone mineralization [40]. This may be why exercise is an effective therapy against postmenopausal osteoporosis. Leukemia inhibitory factor is released during exercise and stimulates muscle growth and regeneration, perhaps by stem cell renewal [41]. Exercise causes the release of fibroblast growth factor 21 (FGF21) that stimulates tissue repair [42].

Lack of exercise has negative effects on the body. Myostatin released by unused muscles decreases muscle size [43], which will decrease insulin clearance. This may lead to fat accumulation.

6. OBESITY

Obesity in adults leads to visceral fat and perivascular fat accumulation [3]. Visceral fat and perivascular fat differ from subdermal fat because visceral and perivascular fat cells secrete adipokines that are inflammatory proteins and toxic lipids [3].

Adipotoxicity occurs during obesity which involves the release of ceramide and toxic amounts of endocannabinoids. Ceramide release into the blood causes inducible nitric oxide synthase (iNOS) dysfunction, damages the kidney and increases blood pressure [44]. Ceramide is critically important since 50% of US adults have heart disease, according to the American Heart Association.

Endocannabinoids such as anandamide and 2-arachidonoyl glycerol are arachidonic acid-derived lipids that mediate the endogenous cannabinoid system in the body by binding to cannabinoid and other receptors. They are normally made in small amounts as needed and in the locations where they are needed. However, the synthesis of endocannabinoids increases inappropriately in obesity. Endocannabinoids increase inflammatory adipokine synthesis [45], stimulate appetite, cause pleasurable feelings and decrease pain. Pain relief is mediated through transient receptor potential cation channels of the vanilloid type (TRPV).

The adipokines leptin and resistin are released into the blood in obesity and increase sympathetic outflow from the brain, causing an autonomic imbalance that increases blood pressure [46]. These blood-born proteins interact with brain regions that are not entirely protected by a blood-brain barrier. High blood pressure can damage the heart leading to congestive heart failure.

6.1. Cancer is promoted by obesity [47, 48], which may involve toll-like receptor (TLR) stimulation by toxic lipids [49] and adipokines [50]. Obesity itself may not cause cancer. But a toxic diet can cause cancer.

6.2. Atherosclerosis is caused by adipokines [3, 51 - 54]. In summary, leptin and visfatin damage arterial walls and cause defects (Table 2). This stimulates the adhesion of platelets, neutrophils and monocytes due to TNFα, resistin and C-reactive protein that stimulate adhesion protein synthesis. Neutrophils induce inflammation by releasing leukotrienes and other inflammatory compounds. Leukotrienes activate TRP channels in endothelial cells, which may cause inflammation. Activation of monocytes and neutrophils causes radical oxygen formation due to the effects of visfatin and leptin. These oxygen radicals oxidize LDL-C, which is taken up by macrophages making foam cells and plaque.

Table 2. Effects of visceral fat on arteries and heart.

Protein factor	Receptor	Pharmacology
Leptin	LEP-R	Neutrophil, monocyte, platelet adhesion and activation
Visfatin	TLR-4	Neutrophil, monocyte, platelet adhesion, matrix metalloproteinase activation, plaque instability
TNFα	TNFR1 and 2	Neutrophil, monocyte, platelet adhesion
Resistin	CAP-1	Increases LDL, monocyte and neutrophil stimulation
C-reactive protein	FcgammaRI and FcgammaRIIa	Increases adhesion protein release by leukocytes, matrix metalloproteinase activation, plaque instability
PDGF	PDGF-R	Smooth muscle proliferation
Angiotensin 2	ATR1 and ATR2	Smooth muscle proliferation
HB-EGF like growth factor	Heparan sulfate proteoglycans, EGF-R	Smooth muscle proliferation

Smooth muscle cell proliferation occurs due to PDGF, angiotensin II and heparin-binding epidermal growth factors like growth factor (HB-EGF), which are all adipokines. Eventually, plaque instability results due to C-reactive protein and visfatin-induced matrix metalloproteinase activity in macrophages. This may lead to emboli, heart attacks, and strokes.

6.3. Type 2 diabetes is caused by adipokines and toxic lipids (Table 3). Fat accumulates in every organ, including muscle, decreasing insulin clearance and sensitivity. Insulin resistance is the basis of type 2 diabetes. The US population is currently suffering from diabetes in epic proportions. According to the Centers for Disease Control, at least 10% of US adults have type 2 diabetes as of 2017.

Table 3. Effects of visceral fat on glucose metabolism.

Factor	Receptor	Pharmacology
Endocannabinoids	CB1, CB2, TRPV	Inflammatory adipokine release
Ceramide	IR, iNOS,	IR dysfunction, pancreatic β cell toxicity
Resistin	CAP-1	IR dysfunction

(Table 3) cont.....

Factor	Receptor	Pharmacology
RELMs	Unknown	IR dysfunction
Visfatin	TLR-4	Long term IR dysfunction
IL-6	IL6R	Long term IR dysfunction
TNFα	TNFR1 and 2	Long term IR dysfunction

A mechanism has been proposed for how obesity causes type 2 diabetes [52, 53, 54]. Endocannabinoids are abundant in visceral fat and are released into the blood. They decrease adiponectin, increase visfatin, TNFα and other inflammatory adipokine releases. Ceramide levels are high in visceral fat and is released into the blood. It inhibits insulin receptor (IR) phosphorylation causing dysfunction. Ceramide also induces iNOS that dysfunctions making oxygen radicals that destroy pancreatic β cells. Resistance of the insulin receptor involves the inflammatory adipokines resistin, resistin-like molecules (RELMs) and ceramide lipotoxicity. Long-term dysfunction of insulin receptors involves the adipokines visfatin, IL-6 and TNFα.

6.4. Osteoarthritis is caused by adipokines and toxic lipids as described in a recent mechanism [3, 57 - 59]. Endocannabinoids decrease adiponectin and increase inflammatory adipokines. However, rheumatoid arthritis patients have high adiponectin levels, perhaps as a compensatory mechanism. According to the Centers for Disease Control, 12% of US adults had osteoarthritis in 2016, compared to 8% in the 1980s. The increase in arthritis in the US is abundantly obvious based on the explosion of prescriptions for oral opioids. The inflammatory adipokine leptin, increases and activates macrophages, T cells, and chondrocytes. This causes these cells to produce oxygen radicals, prostaglandins, chemokines and cytokines that are inflammatory to the bone and cartilage. Inflammation develops and is further increased when macrophages become osteoclasts due to the release of colony-stimulating factor-1 (CSF-1) from fibroblasts. Osteoclasts cause bone erosion and osteoporosis. TNFα is involved in the stimulation of CSF-1 production. Neutrophils are activated by leptin and visfatin, which secrete leukotrienes and other inflammatory factors. Macrophages secrete resistin that induces TNFα and IL-6 in a vicious cycle (Table **4**).

6.5. The Immune system is altered by obesity [60]. Adipokines, such as leptin, cause a dysregulation of the immune system that may increase autoimmune disorders such as rheumatoid arthritis. In obesity, Natural killer (NK) cells decrease and are inactivated, dendritic cells are activated and become more abundant, CD4+ T cells decrease and Treg cells decrease. This immune dysregulation alters the ability of patients to fight infections. The CDC lists obesity as a risk factor for COVID-19 complications and death.

7. ALCOHOL CONSUMPTION

Alcohol is addictive, an obesogen, shifts liver cellular metabolism toward NADH synthesis and away from glycogen synthesis. As a result, fatty acid synthesis increases. This can lead to visceral fat accumulation and fatty liver disease. Alcohol is metabolized by alcohol dehydrogenase to produce acetaldehyde and NADH [61]. Acetaldehyde is metabolized by aldehyde dehydrogenase to produce acetic acid and NADH [61]. NADH shifts the cell to a more reduced state than normal. Glycogen is required for energy during exercise. The depletion of glycogen and accumulation of fat decreases the ability of people to be physically active. Cancer cells, and perhaps precancerous cells, have high alcohol dehydrogenase activity and low aldehyde dehydrogenase activity [61], suggesting that acetaldehyde induction of cancer may explain some of the cancer-causing activity of alcohol.

Alcohol activates peroxisome proliferator-activated receptor γ, thereby altering lipid metabolism [62]. Part of this activity involves enhanced NADH levels which inhibit sirtuin 1 activity. Sirtuin 1 deacetylates and deactivates peroxisome proliferator-activated receptor γ. This alters lipid metabolism resulting in fat accumulation. That is why alcohol is an obesogen.

8. STRESS

Stress is the body's method of reacting to a challenge [63]. The body has several mechanisms to choose from in this response. The autonomic nervous system can regulate blood pressure, heart rate, bronchodilation, glycogenolysis, and gluconeogenesis and comprises the sympathetic nervous system and the parasympathetic nervous system. Balancing these nervous systems, which both respond to stress, is vital for the maintenance of normal health. The hypothalamic-pituitary-adrenal axis also responds to stress and regulates cortisol, vasopressin, and other hormones. Cortisol is immunosuppressive. Activation of the sympathetic nervous system, such as by stress, decreases the innate immune system, making infections more difficult to combat [64]. Epinephrine released by this nervous system can suppress inflammatory cytokine releases, such as IL-10, TNFα, IL-6, and IL-8. The brain regulates the sympathetic and parasympathetic nervous systems and balances these two nervous systems.

Stress promotes alcohol drinking, smoking and overeating [65 - 67]. In addition, glucocorticoids released during stress promote the deposition of visceral fat. Stress is very important in obesity and obesity-related diseases.

Table 4. Effects of visceral fat on arthritis.

Factor	Receptor	Pharmacology
Leptin	LEP-R	Activates macrophages, neutrophils, T cells and chondrocytes. Macrophages secrete TNFα that increases resistin, IL-6 and become osteoclasts. Neutrophils secrete leukotrienes that cause long term inflammation.
TNFα	TNFR1 and 2	CSF-1 production, macrophages become osteoclasts and make oxygen radicals
Visfatin	TLR-4	Neutrophil activation and leukotriene release
Resistin	CAP-1	Released by macrophages, induces TNFα and IL-6 release from fibroblasts

9. BLUE ZONES

The people who live to be over 100 years old have several things in common [68]. They walk and move daily as part of their normal daily routines. They have a purpose for living. They know how to decrease the effects of stress in their lives. They know to eat only 80% of what they could eat. They eat mostly vegetable, fruit and bean-based diets. They drink no more than 1 or 2 glasses of wine daily. They belong to faith-based communities. They put their families before themselves. They have supportive social circles. This is living in balance.

CONCLUSIONS

Modern medicine is faced with many diseases that cannot be cured, such as hypertension, heart disease, arthritis and type 2 diabetes. All of these diseases are managed with drug therapy. This makes the drug companies rich and endangers patients' lives since these drugs all have toxicity problems. These diseases can all be prevented and cured by living in balance. The Framingham studies and other studies have shown that losing weight and exercising can cure these diseases. Cancer can frequently be cured. However, it would be best to prevent cancer. Living in balance can prevent cancer.

REFERENCES

[1]   Adams J. The balanced diet for you and the planet. La Crescenta: Abedus Press 2014.

[2]   Adams JD, Lien EJ. The traditional and scientific bases for traditional Chinese medicine: communication between traditional practitioners, physicians and scientists. In: Adams JD, Lien EJ, Eds. Traditional Chinese medicine – scientific basis for its use. London: Royal Society of Chemistry 2013; pp. 1-10.
[http://dx.doi.org/10.1039/9781849737852-00001]

[3]   Adams JD, Lien E, Parker K. Extracellular and Intracellular Signaling – a New Approach to Diseases and Treatments.Extracellular and intracellular signaling. London: Royal Society of Chemistry 2011; pp. 1-9.
[http://dx.doi.org/10.1039/9781849733434-00001]

[4]   Adams JD. Risk factors for obesity. In: Peplow P, Young T, Adams JD, Eds. Cardiovascular and metabolic disease scientific discoveries and new therapies. London: Royal Society of Chemistry 2015; pp. 59-65.
[http://dx.doi.org/10.1039/9781782622390-00059]

[5]   Mahmood SS, Levy D, Vasan RS, Wang TJ. The Framingham Heart Study and the epidemiology of cardiovascular disease: a historical perspective. Lancet 2014; 383(9921): 999-1008.
[http://dx.doi.org/10.1016/S0140-6736(13)61752-3] [PMID: 24084292]

[6]   Li Y, Schoufour J, Wang DD, *et al.* Healthy lifestyle and life expectancy free of cancer, cardiovascular disease, and type 2 diabetes: prospective cohort study. BMJ 2020; 368: l6669.
[http://dx.doi.org/10.1136/bmj.l6669] [PMID: 31915124]

[7]   Chan DS, Lau R, Aune D, *et al.* Red and processed meat and colorectal cancer incidence: meta-analysis of prospective studies. PLoS One 2011; 6(6): e20456.
[http://dx.doi.org/10.1371/journal.pone.0020456] [PMID: 21674008]

[8]   Liu F, Liu Y, Sun X, *et al.* Race- and sex-specific association between alcohol consumption and hypertension in 22 cohort studies: A systematic review and meta-analysis. Nutr Metab Cardiovasc Dis 2020; 30(8): 1249-59.
[http://dx.doi.org/10.1016/j.numecd.2020.03.018] [PMID: 32446870]

[9]   McCullough ML, Feskanich D, Stampfer MJ, *et al.* Diet quality and major chronic disease risk in men and women: moving toward improved dietary guidance. Am J Clin Nutr 2002; 76(6): 1261-71.
[http://dx.doi.org/10.1093/ajcn/76.6.1261] [PMID: 12450892]

[10]   Sachs KV, Harnke B, Mehler PS, Krantz MJ. Cardiovascular complications of anorexia nervosa: A systematic review. Int J Eat Disord 2016; 49(3): 238-48.
[http://dx.doi.org/10.1002/eat.22481] [PMID: 26710932]

[11]   Weber DD, Aminzadeh-Gohari S, Tulipan J, Catalano L, Feichtinger RG, Kofler B. Ketogenic diet in the treatment of cancer - Where do we stand? Mol Metab 2020; 33: 102-21.
[http://dx.doi.org/10.1016/j.molmet.2019.06.026] [PMID: 31399389]

[12]   Sherrier M, Li H. The impact of keto-adaptation on exercise performance and the role of metabolic-regulating cytokines. Am J Clin Nutr 2019; 110(3): 562-73.
[http://dx.doi.org/10.1093/ajcn/nqz145] [PMID: 31347659]

[13]   Warren GW, Cummings KM. Tobacco and lung cancer: risks, trends, and outcomes in patients with cancer. Am Soc Clin Oncol Educ Book 2013; 359-64.
[http://dx.doi.org/10.14694/EdBook_AM.2013.33.359] [PMID: 23714547]

[14]   Wang TW, Asman K, Gentzke AS, *et al.* Tobacco product use among adults - United States, 2017. MMWR Morb Mortal Wkly Rep 2018; 67(44): 1225-32.
[http://dx.doi.org/10.15585/mmwr.mm6744a2] [PMID: 30408019]

[15]   Bruijnzeel AW. Neuropeptide systems and new treatments for nicotine addiction. Psychopharmacology (Berl) 2017; 234(9-10): 1419-37.
[http://dx.doi.org/10.1007/s00213-016-4513-5] [PMID: 28028605]

[16]   Vazquez-Padron RI, Mateu D, Rodriguez-Menocal L, Wei Y, Webster KA, Pham SM. Novel role of Egr-1 in nicotine-related neointimal formation. Cardiovasc Res 2010; 88(2): 296-303.
[http://dx.doi.org/10.1093/cvr/cvq213] [PMID: 20615913]

[17]   Di Stefano R, Barsotti MC, Felice F, *et al.* Smoking and endothelial progenitor cells: a revision of literature. Curr Pharm Des 2010; 16(23): 2559-66.
[http://dx.doi.org/10.2174/138161210792062939] [PMID: 20550506]

[18]   Kaur J, Reddy K, Balakumar P. The novel role of fenofibrate in preventing nicotine- and sodium arsenite-induced vascular endothelial dysfunction in the rat. Cardiovasc Toxicol 2010; 10(3): 227-38.
[http://dx.doi.org/10.1007/s12012-010-9086-7] [PMID: 20694523]

[19]   Xie YH, Wang SW, Zhang Y, Edvinsson L, Xu CB. Up-regulation of G-protein-coupled receptors for endothelin and thromboxane by lipid-soluble smoke particles in renal artery of rat. Basic Clin Pharmacol Toxicol 2010; 107(4): 803-12.
[http://dx.doi.org/10.1111/j.1742-7843.2010.00585.x] [PMID: 20406207]

[20]   Adams J, Wong M, Villasenor E. Healing with medicinal plants of the west – cultural and scientific basis for their use fourth edition. La Crescenta: Abedus Press 2020.

[21]   Lobelo F, Rohm Young D, Sallis R, *et al.* Routine Assessment and Promotion of Physical Activity in Healthcare Settings: A Scientific Statement From the American Heart Association. Circulation 2018; 137(18): e495-522.
[http://dx.doi.org/10.1161/CIR.0000000000000559] [PMID: 29618598]

[22]   Johnsgard K. The exercise prescription for depression and anxiety. New York: Hachette Books 1989.

[23]   Moore SC, Patel AV, Matthews CE, *et al.* Leisure time physical activity of moderate to vigorous intensity and mortality: a large pooled cohort analysis. PLoS Med 2012; 9(11): e1001335.
[http://dx.doi.org/10.1371/journal.pmed.1001335] [PMID: 23139642]

[24]   Fries JF, Singh G, Morfeld D, Hubert HB, Lane NE, Brown BW Jr. Running and the development of disability with age. Ann Intern Med 1994; 121(7): 502-9.
[http://dx.doi.org/10.7326/0003-4819-121-7-199410010-00005] [PMID: 8067647]

[25]   Liemohn W. Exercise and arthritis. Exercise and the back. Rheum Dis Clin North Am 1990; 16(4): 945-70.
[http://dx.doi.org/10.1016/S0889-857X(21)00917-0] [PMID: 2087586]

[26]   Panush RS. Does exercise cause arthritis? Long-term consequences of exercise on the musculoskeletal system. Rheum Dis Clin North Am 1990; 16(4): 827-36.
[http://dx.doi.org/10.1016/S0889-857X(21)00910-8] [PMID: 2087579]

[27]   Elward K, Larson E, Wagner E. Factors associated with regular aerobic exercise in an elderly population. J Am Board Fam Pract 1992; 5(5): 467-74.
[PMID: 1414447]

[28]   Ward MM, Hubert HB, Shi H, Bloch DA. Physical disability in older runners: prevalence, risk factors, and progression with age. J Gerontol A Biol Sci Med Sci 1995; 50(2): M70-7.
[http://dx.doi.org/10.1093/gerona/50A.2.M70] [PMID: 7874592]

[29]   Fries JF, Singh G, Morfeld D, O'Driscoll P, Hubert H. Relationship of running to musculoskeletal pain with age. A six-year longitudinal study. Arthritis Rheum 1996; 39(1): 64-72.
[http://dx.doi.org/10.1002/art.1780390109] [PMID: 8546740]

[30]   Bruce B, Fries JF, Lubeck DP. Aerobic exercise and its impact on musculoskeletal pain in older adults: a 14 year prospective, longitudinal study. Arthritis Res Ther 2005; 7(6): R1263-70.
[http://dx.doi.org/10.1186/ar1825] [PMID: 16277679]

[31]   Heath GW, Gavin JR III, Hinderliter JM, Hagberg JM, Bloomfield SA, Holloszy JO. Effects of exercise and lack of exercise on glucose tolerance and insulin sensitivity. J Appl Physiol 1983; 55(2): 512-7.
[http://dx.doi.org/10.1152/jappl.1983.55.2.512] [PMID: 6352578]

[32]   Ceddia RB, Somwar R, Maida A, Fang X, Bikopoulos G, Sweeney G. Globular adiponectin increases GLUT4 translocation and glucose uptake but reduces glycogen synthesis in rat skeletal muscle cells. Diabetologia 2005; 48(1): 132-9.
[http://dx.doi.org/10.1007/s00125-004-1609-y] [PMID: 15619075]

[33]   Pedersen BK, Steensberg A, Schjerling P. Muscle-derived interleukin-6: possible biological effects. J Physiol 2001; 536(Pt 2): 329-37.
[http://dx.doi.org/10.1111/j.1469-7793.2001.0329c.xd] [PMID: 11600669]

[34]   Barra NG, Palanivel R, Denou E, *et al.* Interleukin-15 modulates adipose tissue by altering

mitochondrial mass and activity. PLoS One 2014; 9(12): e114799.
[http://dx.doi.org/10.1371/journal.pone.0114799] [PMID: 25517731]

[35]   Matthews VB, Aström MB, Chan MH, *et al.* Brain-derived neurotrophic factor is produced by skeletal muscle cells in response to contraction and enhances fat oxidation *via* activation of AMP-activated protein kinase. Diabetologia 2009; 52(7): 1409-18.
[http://dx.doi.org/10.1007/s00125-009-1364-1] [PMID: 19387610]

[36]   Liu PZ, Nusslock R. Exercise-Mediated Neurogenesis in the Hippocampus *via* BDNF. Front Neurosci 2018; 12: 52.
[http://dx.doi.org/10.3389/fnins.2018.00052] [PMID: 29467613]

[37]   Seldin MM, Peterson JM, Byerly MS, Wei Z, Wong GW. Myonectin (CTRP15), a novel myokine that links skeletal muscle to systemic lipid homeostasis. J Biol Chem 2012; 287(15): 11968-80.
[http://dx.doi.org/10.1074/jbc.M111.336834] [PMID: 22351773]

[38]   Kanzleiter T, Rath M, Görgens SW, *et al.* The myokine decorin is regulated by contraction and involved in muscle hypertrophy. Biochem Biophys Res Commun 2014; 450(2): 1089-94.
[http://dx.doi.org/10.1016/j.bbrc.2014.06.123] [PMID: 24996176]

[39]   Boström P, Wu J, Jedrychowski MP, *et al.* A PGC1-α-dependent myokine that drives brown-fat-like development of white fat and thermogenesis. Nature 2012; 481(7382): 463-8.
[http://dx.doi.org/10.1038/nature10777] [PMID: 22237023]

[40]   Termine JD, Kleinman HK, Whitson SW, Conn KM, McGarvey ML, Martin GR. Osteonectin, a bone-specific protein linking mineral to collagen. Cell 1981; 26(1 Pt 1): 99-105.
[http://dx.doi.org/10.1016/0092-8674(81)90037-4] [PMID: 7034958]

[41]   Nicola NA, Babon JJ. Leukemia inhibitory factor (LIF). Cytokine Growth Factor Rev 2015; 26(5): 533-44.
[http://dx.doi.org/10.1016/j.cytogfr.2015.07.001] [PMID: 26187859]

[42]   Xie T, Leung PS. Fibroblast growth factor 21: a regulator of metabolic disease and health span. Am J Physiol Endocrinol Metab 2017; 313(3): E292-302.
[http://dx.doi.org/10.1152/ajpendo.00101.2017] [PMID: 28559437]

[43]   Jespersen JG, Nedergaard A, Andersen LL, Schjerling P, Andersen JL. Myostatin expression during human muscle hypertrophy and subsequent atrophy: increased myostatin with detraining. Scand J Med Sci Sports 2011; 21(2): 215-23.
[http://dx.doi.org/10.1111/j.1600-0838.2009.01044.x] [PMID: 19903317]

[44]   Won JS, Im YB, Khan M, Singh AK, Singh I. The role of neutral sphingomyelinase produced ceramide in lipopolysaccharide-mediated expression of inducible nitric oxide synthase. J Neurochem 2004; 88(3): 583-93.
[http://dx.doi.org/10.1046/j.1471-4159.2003.02165.x] [PMID: 14720208]

[45]   Ge Q, Maury E, Rycken L, *et al.* Endocannabinoids regulate adipokine production and the immune balance of omental adipose tissue in human obesity. Int J Obes 2013; 37(6): 874-80.
[http://dx.doi.org/10.1038/ijo.2012.123] [PMID: 22868830]

[46]   Badoer E, Kosari S, Stebbing MJ. Resistin, an Adipokine with Non-Generalized Actions on Sympathetic Nerve Activity. Front Physiol 2015; 6: 321-33.
[http://dx.doi.org/10.3389/fphys.2015.00321] [PMID: 26617526]

[47]   Paz-Filho G, Lim EL, Wong ML, Licinio J. Associations between adipokines and obesity-related cancer. Front Biosci 2011; 16: 1634-50.
[http://dx.doi.org/10.2741/3810] [PMID: 21196253]

[48]   Booth A, Magnuson A, Fouts J, Foster M. Adipose tissue, obesity and adipokines: role in cancer promotion. Horm Mol Biol Clin Investig 2015; 21(1): 57-74.
[http://dx.doi.org/10.1515/hmbci-2014-0037] [PMID: 25781552]

[49]   Rakoff-Nahoum S, Medzhitov R. Toll-like receptors and cancer. Nat Rev Cancer 2009; 9(1): 57-63.

[http://dx.doi.org/10.1038/nrc2541] [PMID: 19052556]

[50]   Wang SN, Wang ST, Lee KT. The potential interplay of adipokines with toll-like receptors in the development of hepatocellular carcinoma. Gastroenterol Res Pract 2011; 2011: 215986.
       [http://dx.doi.org/10.1155/2011/215986] [PMID: 21960997]

[51]   Ritchie SA, Connell JM. The link between abdominal obesity, metabolic syndrome and cardiovascular disease. Nutr Metab Cardiovasc Dis 2007; 17(4): 319-26.
       [http://dx.doi.org/10.1016/j.numecd.2006.07.005] [PMID: 17110092]

[52]   Alberti KG, Eckel RH, Grundy SM, *et al.* Harmonizing the metabolic syndrome: a joint interim statement of the International Diabetes Federation Task Force on Epidemiology and Prevention; National Heart, Lung, and Blood Institute; American Heart Association; World Heart Federation; International Atherosclerosis Society; and International Association for the Study of Obesity. Circulation 2009; 120: 1640-5.

[53]   Adams J, Parker K. Extracellular and Intracellular Signaling. London: Royal Society of Chemistry 2011.
       [http://dx.doi.org/10.1039/9781849733434]

[54]   Taube A, Schlich R, Sell H, Eckardt K, Eckel J. Inflammation and metabolic dysfunction: links to cardiovascular diseases. Am J Physiol Heart Circ Physiol 2012; 302(11): H2148-65.
       [http://dx.doi.org/10.1152/ajpheart.00907.2011] [PMID: 22447947]

[55]   Walker CG, Zariwala MG, Holness MJ, Sugden MC. Diet, obesity and diabetes: a current update. Clin Sci (Lond) 2007; 112(2): 93-111.
       [http://dx.doi.org/10.1042/CS20060150] [PMID: 17155931]

[56]   Pittas AG, Joseph NA, Greenberg AS. Adipocytokines and insulin resistance. J Clin Endocrinol Metab 2004; 89(2): 447-52.
       [http://dx.doi.org/10.1210/jc.2003-031005] [PMID: 14764746]

[57]   Matias I, Di Marzo V. Endocannabinoids and the control of energy balance. Trends Endocrinol Metab 2007; 18(1): 27-37.
       [http://dx.doi.org/10.1016/j.tem.2006.11.006] [PMID: 17141520]

[58]   Otero M, Lago R, Gomez R, *et al.* Towards a pro-inflammatory and immunomodulatory emerging role of leptin. Rheumatology (Oxford) 2006; 45(8): 944-50.
       [http://dx.doi.org/10.1093/rheumatology/kel157] [PMID: 16720637]

[59]   Senolt L, Housa D, Vernerová Z, *et al.* Resistin in rheumatoid arthritis synovial tissue, synovial fluid and serum. Ann Rheum Dis 2007; 66(4): 458-63.
       [http://dx.doi.org/10.1136/ard.2006.054734] [PMID: 17040961]

[60]   Francisco V, Pino J, Campos-Cabaleiro V, *et al.* Obesity, Fat mass and immune system: role for leptin. Front Physiol 2018; 9: 640.
       [http://dx.doi.org/10.3389/fphys.2018.00640] [PMID: 29910742]

[61]   Jelski W, Szmitkowski M. Alcohol dehydrogenase (ADH) and aldehyde dehydrogenase (ALDH) in the cancer diseases. Clin Chim Acta 2008; 395(1-2): 1-5.
       [http://dx.doi.org/10.1016/j.cca.2008.05.001] [PMID: 18505683]

[62]   Yu JH, Song SJ, Kim A, *et al.* Suppression of PPARγ-mediated monoacylglycerol O-acyltransferase 1 expression ameliorates alcoholic hepatic steatosis. Sci Rep 2016; 6: 29352.
       [http://dx.doi.org/10.1038/srep29352] [PMID: 27404390]

[63]   Goldstein DS, Kopin IJ. Evolution of concepts of stress. Stress 2007; 10(2): 109-20.
       [http://dx.doi.org/10.1080/10253890701288935] [PMID: 17514579]

[64]   Kox M, van Eijk LT, Zwaag J, *et al.* Voluntary activation of the sympathetic nervous system and attenuation of the innate immune response in humans. Proc Natl Acad Sci USA 2014; 111(20): 7379-84.
       [http://dx.doi.org/10.1073/pnas.1322174111] [PMID: 24799686]

[65]   Yau YH, Potenza MN. Stress and eating behaviors. Minerva Endocrinol 2013; 38(3): 255-67.
        [PMID: 24126546]

[66]   Vasse RM, Nijhuis FJ, Kok G. Associations between work stress, alcohol consumption and sickness
        absence. Addiction 1998; 93(2): 231-41.
        [http://dx.doi.org/10.1046/j.1360-0443.1998.9322317.x] [PMID: 9624724]

[67]   Smokefree.gov, Office on Smoking and Health, National Center for Chronic Disease Prevention and
        Health Promotion, Centers for Disease Control and Prevention. Accessed September 2, 2021.

[68]   Buettner D, Skemp S. Blue zones: Lessons from the world's longest lived. Am J Lifestyle Med 2016;
        10(5): 318-21.
        [http://dx.doi.org/10.1177/1559827616637066] [PMID: 30202288]

CHAPTER 2

Spirituality and Balance

Abstract: Most religions teach moderation, which is the balance between excess and deficit. Moderation leads to happiness and good health. Spirituality can teach people to be moderate and motivate people to maintain healthy lifestyles. The Chumash Indian Religion is discussed in detail since balance is an essential component of the religion.

Keywords: African, Buddhism, Christianity, Chumash, Confucianism, Hinduism, Islam, Moderation, Sacred Medicine, Taoism.

1. INTRODUCTION

Patients with chronic diseases are frequently advised to make lifestyle changes such as exercising more and getting rid of excess weight. Healthcare professionals may be less likely to recommend adding spirituality to lifestyle changes. A recent study found that patients with chronic diseases seek more spirituality in their self-management [1]. This spirituality can be good, such as adding inner strength. Spirituality can also negatively affect patients who experience inner battles, feelings of guilt and becoming a victim. Spiritual leaders should be ready to counsel patients experiencing negative effects.

2. CHRISTIANITY

Balance is a concept that appears in most religions. Balance is discussed several times in the Bible. Ecclesiastes 3 describes the process of balance in the world. "For everything, there is a season, and a time for every matter under heaven: a time to be born, and a time to die; a time to plant, and a time to pluck up what is planted; a time to kill, and a time to heal; a time to break down, and a time to build up; a time to weep, and a time to laugh; a time to mourn, and a time to dance; a time to cast away stones, and a time to gather stones together; a time to embrace, and a time to refrain from embracing; a time to seek, and a time to lose; a time to keep, and a time to cast away; a time to tear, and a time to sew; a time to keep silence, and a time to speak; a time to love, and a time to hate; a time for war, and a time for peace." These are traditional principles of balance that apply today also.

In traditional times, obesity was considered out of balance. Proverbs 11 describes this "A false balance is an abomination to the Lord, but a just weight is his delight." This can also be understood as using a balance to weigh and depending on a just weight for accuracy. Second, Timothy teaches in verse 1 "For God gave us a spirit not of fear but power and love and self-control." We are advised to practice self-control which is part of our spirits. Third John verse 1 tells us that good health and spirituality are linked. "Beloved, I pray that all may go well with you and that you may be in good health, as it goes well with your soul." Self-control and maintaining a just weight are tied to our spirituality.

Spirituality is encouraged in the Bible as a way of achieving balance and a good life. First John 1 admonishes, "Do not love the world or the things in the world. If anyone loves the world, the love of the Father is not in him. All that is in the world—the desires of the flesh and the desires of the eyes and pride in possessions—is not from the Father but the world. And the world is passing away along with its desires, but whoever does the will of God abides forever." In other words, being spiritual and avoiding the desires of the flesh, like over-eating, are helpful to us.

First Corinthians 6 tells us how important our bodies are "Or do you not know that your body is a temple of the Holy Spirit within you, whom you have from God? You are not your own." In other words, living a healthy life in balance is a spiritual necessity since the Holy Spirit dwells within us.

The Bible also encourages exercise and hard work as in Matthew 11 "Come to me, all who labor and are heavily laden, and I will give you rest. Take my yoke upon you, and learn from me, for I am gentle and lowly in heart, and you will find rest for your souls. For my yoke is easy, and my burden is light." We are told to find rest, replenishment, in spirituality after working hard.

We are also admonished that God will judge us as in Proverbs 16 "A just balance and scales are the Lord's; all the weights in the bag are his work." Job 31 has a similar passage "Let me be weighed in a just balance, and let God know my integrity!" Just as God judges us, our bodies also tell us the truth about how well we live in balance. Chronic diseases, such as heart disease, type 2 diabetes and arthritis, afflict us when we are not in balance.

3. ISLAMIC FAITH

In the Quran, balance is mentioned several times. Transgression means the loss of balance. 40 Forgiver 28 "Truly God guides not one who transgresses and lies." God encourages balance and guides those in balance. Ash-Shura, Chapter #42 tells us that "It is God who has sent down the Book (the Quran) in truth, and the balance (*i.e.* to act justly)." God tells us "Thus, we have made you a justly balanced community that you will be witnesses over the people" Surat Al-Baqarah 2:143. It is important for the community to be in balance. This is a crucial issue in traditional communities where only a certain number of people can be supported by the social structure. In order for people to survive, the community must be in balance.

"Every praiseworthy characteristic has two blameworthy poles. Generosity is the middle between miserliness and extravagance. Courage is the middle between cowardice and recklessness. Humanity has been commanded to avoid every such blameworthy trait" Lisan al-Arab 15/209. Balance in personality characteristics is as important as balance in health characteristics. Moderation is encouraged and helps people stay in balance. A man who fasted all day and prayed all night was told, "Do not do so. Fast and break your fast, pray in the night and sleep. Verily, your body has a right over you, your eyes have a right over you, and your wife has a right over you" Sahih Bukhari 4903. This shows the importance of fasting and praying to maintain balance. Fasting can help maintain the balance of the body. "You have a duty to your Lord, you have a duty to your body, and you have a duty to your family, so you should give each one its rights" Sahih Bukhari 1867. Spirituality and maintaining good health are important to living a balanced life [2].

4. HINDUISM

The Maitrayaniya Upanishads teach us "those who realize the Self enter into the peace that brings complete self-control and perfect patience. They see themselves in everyone and everyone in themselves." The Self is Brahman (God), who lives inside each person's heart. Therefore, spirituality and bodily health are intertwined.

Prajapati, the Lord of all creatures, divided himself into five pieces and entered into all living creatures. Prana is upward breath, inhaling and taking in energy. Apana is downward breath, exhaling and using energy. Vyana is the circulation of energy that maintains a balance between Prana and Apana. Samana is exertion and the digestion of nutrients to fuel exertion. Udana is the energy of the brain and throat in communication and processing thoughts. The Lord of all creatures helps us in five ways to be healthy and in balance.

Hinduism teaches men to be in balance with nature. Polluting water, air, and the ocean is discouraged [3]. We are taught that God lives in the air, water, fire, trees, and herbs. Men should have reverence for the places God lives.

5. BUDDHISM

The middle way is taught in Buddhism, which is living a practical life without extremes of self-denial or self-indulgence. This involves a mental attitude of balance, detachment and impartiality. We are taught that acceptance balances change [4]. In fact, mental attitude is important to balance [5]. Living in the middle way is essential when choosing what to eat, wear, what to say, where to go and all aspects of life.

His Holiness, the Dalai Lama, has written, "Today there is an overemphasis on the external world. Science has rapidly extended our understanding of external phenomena, and technological advances have contributed to improved health and physical comfort. Yet even in the most developed countries, we do not find a corresponding increase in peace and happiness; if anything, there is greater anxiety and stress. Fear stimulates the need for terrifyingly destructive weapons systems, while greed gives rise to damage and pollution of the environment, putting the very existence of humanity at risk" [6].

Clearly, understanding and technological advances should be balanced with peace and happiness. Anxiety, stress, and greed must be balanced with kindness in order to avoid damaging ourselves and our environment.

6. TAOISM

Laozi wrote in the Tao Te Ching "The great Way (Tao) is easy, yet people prefer the side paths. Be aware when things are out of balance. Stay centered within the Tao." The Tao is the Way to govern, to work and to live in general. Everything comes from nothing and will return to nothing in an eternal cycle. "As it acts in the world, the Tao is like the bending of a bow. The top is bent downward. The bottom is bent up. It adjusts excess and deficiency so that there is a perfect balance. It takes from what is too much and gives to what is not enough." The Tao balances the world without effort from mankind. We are taught that the efforts of man can make the world out of balance. The adverse effects of man are obvious in an overpopulated, over-polluted and over-exploited world. Perhaps if mankind lived in the Taoist manner, we would not suffer from pandemics like COVID-19, which are spread rapidly in an overpopulated society.

7. CONFUCIANISM

There must be a balance between yin and yang in order for heaven, the world and our bodies to be in balance [7]. Yin is feminine and cold. Yang is masculine and hot. Yin and yang depend on chi, the vital energy that flows in heaven, the world and our bodies. Similarly, chi comes from yin and yang. Clearly, there must be men and women in order for children to be born. But the world must have a balance where the population does not exceed the ability of the world to provide for people. There is a similar balance for heaven. When the world and our bodies are in balance, heaven is in balance.

Our bodies must be in balance for health [8 - 11]. Each of us has yin and yang in our bodies. Blood flowing in our arteries brings heat to our organs, yang. Lack of blood flow, yin, makes us feel cold. Excessive blood flow is involved in hypertension, too much yang, and can be treated by using antihypertensive agents, yin. However, health can be restored and hypertension can be cured by living in balance [8 - 11].

Chi is the flow of information in the body due to signaling processes, intracellular and extracellular [8, 10]. The use of agonists, yang, and antagonists, yin, for various receptors regulates the flow of information into the cell and out of the cell, chi. This flow of information, chi, is critical for health and balance. Intracellular signals include cAMP, G proteins, NO, Ca^{+2} and other information. Extracellular signals are adipokines, endocannabinoids, prostaglandins, some hormones, osmotic pressure, blood pressure and other signals.

8. TRADITIONAL AFRICAN RELIGIONS

Currently, only 8% of Africans practice traditional religions, such as Vodun. The Vodun religion is practiced by several million people in West Africa, including Benin, Togo, Nigeria and Ghana. Christianity and the Islamic religion have displaced traditional religions. There is very little written about traditional African religions by Africans who actually practice the religions. The majority of the writing comes from Christians. One of the precepts of some African religions is animism, all of God's creations have souls, including trees, rocks, water, animals and man [12].

In the Vodun religion, the sun is male while the moon is female. They exist in a balance to provide the right amount of heat and cold to the world and its people. The sun also provides energy and strength. The moon provides peace, fertility and rain. When the world and its people are in balance, heaven is in balance.

It is interesting that fertility and strength are seen as opposing states in the human body. It is known from female athletes that a strong body with a body fat composition below about 12% tends to be infertile. This is not true of men.

In the Caribbean, Vodun is called Vodou or Voodoo and is practiced by several million people in Jamaica, Haiti, the Dominican Republic, Brazil, and the US. The Voodoo religion combines Vodun and Roman Catholic beliefs and was created by African slaves. The Voodoo religion has served the slaves and their descendants for several hundred years and helped them live in balance. This balance involves the worship of Iwa, Gods, that can be hot or cold, good or subversive.

Malevolence is seen as a normal part of human society that balances good. There are Vodou priests, Bokors, who practice a malevolent ritual to determine the truth. The person being accused of lying is administered a medicine. If the person tells the truth, the person survives. If the person lies, the person becomes a zombie [13]. The medicine administered contains ash, fat and *Datura stramonium*, which is called zombie cucumber in Haiti. This preparation is rubbed onto the abdomen. The ash is alkaline and converts scopolamine from the *D. stramonium* into a free base that rapidly crosses the skin. Scopolamine penetrates into the brain, inhibits muscarinic receptors, inhibits respiration and induces a dream state. Inhibition of respiration can make the person appear dead. The dream state will be discussed more under the Chumash religion. The person may require hours or even a couple of days to recover from the dream state. The person is then considered dead by the community and may be sold into slavery by the Bokor.

9. CHUMASH INDIAN RELIGION

The author was trained for 14 years by a Chumash Indian Healer/Priest, Cecilia Garcia, who was one of the few people in the state of California to actually practice the Chumash Indian Religion. My teacher and I wrote a book and several articles that discuss the Chumash Indian Religion [2, 14, 15]. My teacher was the only person I have met who went through the rite of passage with *Datura wrightii* (Fig. **1**). My teacher died in 2012. I continue her tradition of healing and teaching Chumash healing and the Chumash Religion.

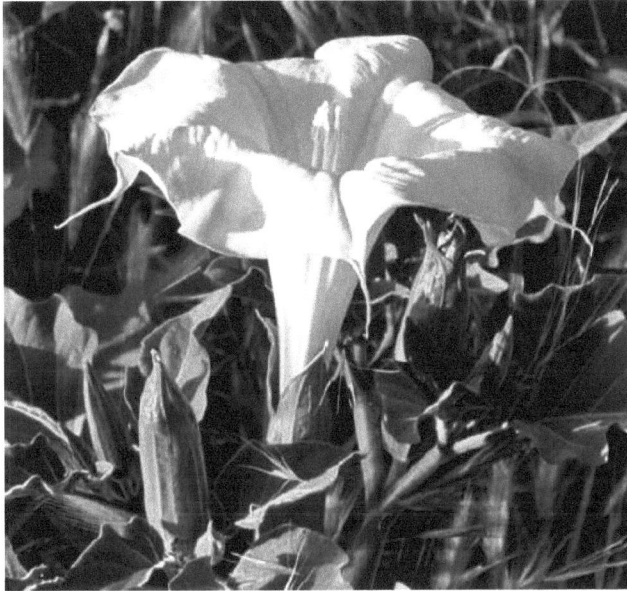

Fig. (1). Datura wrightii, Momoy, used in Sacred Ceremony and medicinally. Photograph by J Adams.

The Chumash Indians' traditional land is coastal Southern California from Malibu to San Luis Obispo and inland for several miles. They have been in California for several thousand years and continue to live in California today.

9.1. Principles

Each person must be productive and help maintain the community. In order to be healthy and productive, each person must live in balance. Balance involves maintaining a strong and thin body. This prevents diseases. Balance also includes spirituality, being a loving family member, being a respectful community member, serving the community, maintaining the environment, and taking no more than what is needed. Living in balance allows the body to heal itself.

One version of the creation story involves balance. All people lived on Santa Cruz Island in the presence of God, Xoy. Some of the people wanted to live on the mainland and be independent of God. God granted their wish. He created a huge flood that separated Santa Cruz Island from the mainland. Then he created a rainbow bridge from Santa Cruz Island to a mountain on the mainland, Mount Piños. He asked the people who wanted to cross the rainbow bridge to promise they would live in balance on the mainland and use the world wisely. The rainbow is a symbol of our promise to God that we will live in balance. He also commanded the people who crossed the bridge not to look down. The people who did look down became frightened and fell into the ocean. God knows how difficult it is for us to follow His commandments. Through His grace, he forgave them and turned them into dolphins so they would not die. Dolphins are the brothers of the Chumash people and remind us that God forgives our sins.

The Chumash Indians believe there is only one God and that all people worship the same God. There are many Angels that help God, such as Sky Coyote, Snilemun, and Sky Eagle, Slo' as explained in interviews with the Chumash people conducted in the early 1900's by a Linguist, John Harrington [16]. It is important to remember that John Harrington was an Atheist and thought the Chumash Religion was ignorant and primitive [17]. As a result, his work has abundant errors.

God helps people keep their balance by giving each of us a spiritual sense [15]. This is similar to what Christians call the Holy Spirit. The spiritual sense helps guide us and keeps us connected with God. We are each born with the spiritual sense. But some people listen better than others.

The community must be in balance. If the community has too few people, they will not survive since not enough food will be gathered to feed them. If the community has too many people, it will be impossible to gather enough food to keep everyone alive, especially during the winter when people go hungry.

The environment must be in balance. If too much is gathered from one area, there will not be enough next year. If too many deer are hunted, or too many fish are collected, there will not be enough next year.

Spirituality must be in balance. In traditional times, every year near the winter solstice, a ceremony was held to pray and ask for guidance. The ceremony included the deer dance and the swordfish dance to show God that the people had hunted and gathered enough but not too much. The Healer/Priests ('Antap) asked for guidance and advice about what would happen next year. Some of the Healer/Priests were experts in astronomy and set very accurate calendars based on the sun, moon and stars [18]. It was critical for the Chumash to know the exact time of the winter solstice so that hunting, fishing, gathering and other schedules could be set. The winter solstice ceremony occurred in an enclosure called the siliyuk [16]. The inside of the enclosure was not visible from the outside due to hanging mats made from tule, *Schoenoplectis acutus*. At the center of the enclosure was an upright log painted with symbols depicting what had happened during the year. This log was burned at the end of the ceremony.

There is a heavenly counterpart to the winter solstice ceremony in which the balance of the world is decided. During the night of the winter solstice, Sky

Coyote and the Sun play a gambling game called peon, in which each player takes turns guessing which hand of the other player holds a concealed stick (Fig. **2**). In the morning, the Sun has to go to work, so the winnings are counted to find out who was the victor. Sky Coyote is a liar and cheater. If Sky Coyote won, the year would be wet and people will survive. Except that Sky Coyote is a trickster and may bring flooding that can harm people. If the Sun is the victor, He takes his winnings in human lives. It will be a hot and dry year in which people will die.

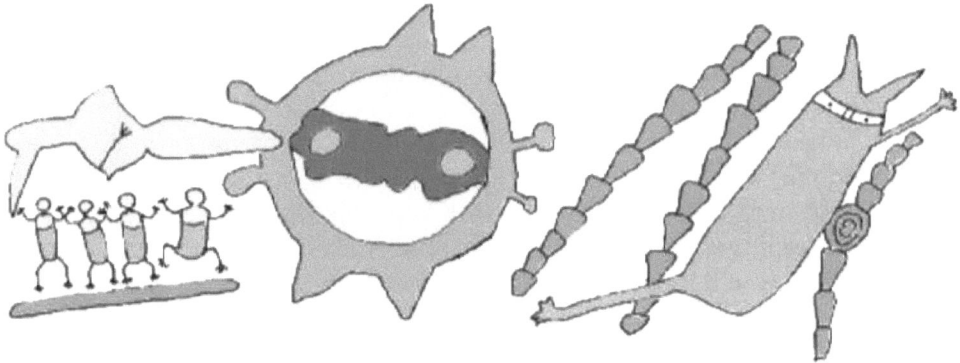

Fig. (2). Sky Coyote and Sun playing peon. Art-work by J Adams.

There were many yearly religious ceremonies and social ceremonies as explained in the Eye of the Flute [19]. The summer solstice ceremony was the time to stop grieving for the dead, in other words, let their souls go to Heaven, Similaqsa. During this ceremony, the people gather in a circle with a fire in the center. Each person who has lost a loved one during the year has a turn at entering into the circle and singing a song for their loved one.

The Healer/Priests were educated at a Medical School in a place now called the Cuddy Valley. After a year of training, they became apprentices to a Healer/Priest for seven years. Then they were ready to be hired by a village or group of villages. Only people chosen by God could become Healer/Priests. Typically the grandchildren of Healer/Priests were chosen. However, anyone could demonstrate they had been chosen by living for a year without eating meat.

My teacher taught me the Chumash people do not believe in the devil. They believe in mischievous spirits called nunasus, which can cause trouble for people. My teacher said "Before the Spanish came, there was no devil in California."

9.2. Spanish Influence

Juan Rodriguez Cabrillo was the first Spaniard to visit California. He sailed along the coast in 1542 and visited Chumash territory, including San Miguel Island [20]. On the Island, he lived among the Chumash people in the winter of 1542 and had intimate relations with at least one woman. He later decided to rape the wife of the Chief (Wot). The Chumash people punished his transgression by smashing his leg. He escaped to Santa Rosa Island, where he died on 3 January 1543 and was buried [21]. The Cabrillo expedition provided an indication of what the Spanish would later do in California. One good result of the expedition was that no gold or silver was found in California which made the Spanish reluctant to return to California.

Saint Junipero Serra, Apostle of California, came to San Diego, California, on 1 July 1769. At that time, there were about 360,00 California Indians. Serra had been a leader of the Spanish Inquisition in Mexico beginning in 1752 and had found evidence of sorcery, witchcraft and devil worship among the Mexican natives. He moved to Baja California in 1768 where the native people were being ravaged by syphilis, probably actually gonorrhea, introduced by the Spanish. Serra suffered from a terrible case of gonorrhea-induced arthritis for the rest of his life.

The Catholics could not find California Indians who were interested in converting to Catholicism. A large part of this problem came from the fact that few if any Spanish learned the California Indian languages and could not adequately communicate with the Indians. The Indians were seen as half-human, half animal because the Indians were about 8 inches taller than the Spanish and had dark skin rather than white skin. In addition, the Indians were called devil worshippers because they did not kneel in front of the cross.

The Catholics founded 5 missions in Chumash Territory, San Fernando (1797), San Buenaventura (1782), Santa Barbara (1786), La Purisima Concepcion (1787) and San Luis Obispo de Tolosa (1772). The Spanish treated the Chumash as animals and devil worshippers, which meant the Indians could be abused and killed as necessary. The Chumash attitude about the Spanish was told to me by a Chumash Elder, Ted Garcia. God sent his Son to the ancestors of the Spanish. They nailed Him to a cross and crucified Him. This made the Chumash reluctant to work with the Spanish since God would someday punish the Spanish for what they had done.

The Spanish collected converts to their missions in a process called child harvesting [22]. The Spanish soldiers and priests would ride their horses into a Chumash village with the cross in front of them. If the Indians did not kneel, the men were shot and killed. The women were captured and raped. The children were kidnapped and enslaved in the missions. The mothers followed their children to the missions. If the fathers were alive, they followed their wives and children to the missions. Child harvesting was practiced at every mission in California.

At the missions, the children lived at the mercy of the priests. In fact, the priests lived like kings in the missions with riches beyond what they would have had in Spain [23]. Since the Chumash were seen as half human, half animal, the priests could have sex with them without breaking their vows of celibacy. Many of the priests were infected with gonorrhea. When a teen-aged girl is infected with gonorrhea, she frequently becomes infertile. Low birth rates were recorded at every California mission. Child harvesting and gonorrhea resulted in the loss of about 120,000 Indian lives in California. Spanish introduced measles and influenza were responsible for some deaths also. This was the first genocide.

9.3. Gold Mining Era

Mexico, and California, became independent of Spain in 1836. The Mexicans secularized the missions. Indians enslaved in the missions were either freed or became enslaved on Mexican ranchos [23]. In 1848, gold was discovered in the American River near Sacramento. Nearly 300,000 gold miners invaded California from Europe and the eastern US to collect and mine gold in two years. California Indians learned to collect gold and were taught by white people from the Sacramento area. When the invaders found Indians collecting gold from the rivers and streams, the white invaders killed the Indians and took the gold [24]. In two years, about 100,000 Indians were killed. Many of these Indians were not involved in gold mining and were killed while living in their traditional ways on their traditional land in the foothills of the Sierra Nevada Mountains. This involved cold-blooded murder of men, women and children. This is the second genocide. There are no records of Chumash people being involved in gold mining at this time.

9.4. United States Influence

In 1850, California was taken from Mexico by US Armed Forces. The US citizens of the state of California decided that California Indians should become extinct [25 - 29]. The US Army came to California to kill Indians. One of the early conquests was the Pomo Indians of Clear Lake. The US Army records of this genocide reveal horrific murders of infants, children, women and men. California Militia units were formed to kill Indians. The Militia men were very well paid, about the same salary that was paid to doctors. For the most part, the Indians did not have guns and were not able to defend themselves against the genocide that proceeded to kill about 120,000 Indians. Indians were hunted from San Diego to past the Oregon border.

Typically, an Indian village was surrounded at night. As the Indians got out of bed in the morning, everyone was killed, men, women and children. Sometimes children were kidnapped and sold into slavery (Fig. **3**). Boys were sold for $30-50. Girls were sold for as much as $200 because they could be used as sex slaves. Since California was a nonslave state, the Indian children could not be called slaves. Instead, they were called apprentices or indentured servants. The third genocide stopped in 1873 when the US citizens of California decided that Indians were extinct.

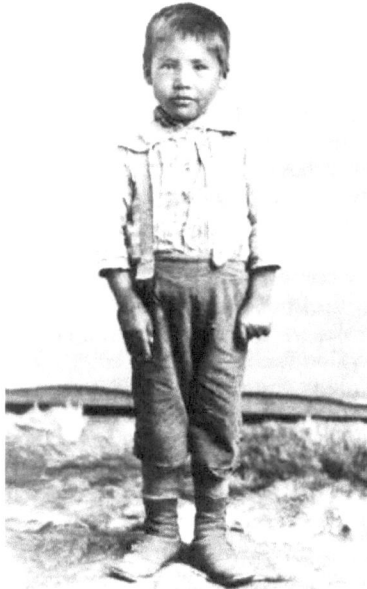

Fig. (3). Apprentice child captured and sold into slavery.

In fact, there were still about 30,000 Indians alive in California. Most of them escaped the genocide by telling white people they were Mexican [23]. This was the truth since the Indians had been born in California when it was part of Mexico. Indians were not allowed to own land or practice their religion. Mexicans could own land. However, the Chumash religion is still illegal in the state of California. It is called felony child endangerment.

10. THE CHUMASH INDIAN RELIGION IS ILLEGAL IN THE US

In October 1855, the US Army visited the Chumash Medical School in the Cuddy

Valley. Any California Indian could be educated to become a healer at the Medical School, not just Chumash people. My teacher's great great grandparents were teachers at the Medical School. The US Army gave them two choices, get out and never come back, or die right now. The teachers left California and went to Mexico. They went where they were needed such as the Chihuahua Mountains near Barbicora, the Mexicali area, Hermosillo or Torreon. On the way out of California, the teachers hid many items of regalia and astronomy in a cave now called Bower's Cave. These items were found by white men and sold to Harvard University.

Most Chumash people today are Catholics and do not want their religion to return to California. They do not want any trouble with the US Army or US officials. Chumash pow-wows occur every year. These are social gatherings, not sacred gatherings.

The Chumash Religion uses Sacred Datura, *Datura wrightii*, called Momoy in Chumash, in the sacred ceremony (Fig. **1**). Momoy contains scopolamine and hyoscyamine [14, 30]. Modern medicine uses these compounds in the clinic. This is considered to be part of good medical practice. However, the Chumash Religion must never use scopolamine and hyoscyamine in religious practice. This is considered ignorant and dangerous.

10.1. First Sacred Dream

In traditional times, the first sacred ceremony each person experienced was the rite of passage. Each child went through a year of instruction by the Healer/Priest and the elders of the village to prepare for adulthood. When a boy needed to become a man or a girl needed to become a woman, the Healer/Priest made a preparation of Momoy and gave it to the mother. The mother announced to the village, "It is time for my son or daughter to die so that a man or woman can be born." The child ingested the preparation. The village sang the Momoy songs to the child so the child would sleep. The Healer/Priest stayed beside the child while the child slept and had Sacred Dreams. The Healer/Priest made sure the child survived even if respiratory depression occurred. Scopolamine penetrates into the brain, inhibits muscarinic receptors in the cerebral cortex, activates pyramidal neurons and allows Sacred Dreams to occur [14, 15]. However, respiratory depression can also occur. During the Sacred Dream the child's spirit went to God. The child was taught by God how to become an adult and was set on the path to the profession God had chosen for the child. If the child agreed with what God had chosen, the child returned to the village and had earned a place in the village.

Each Sacred Dream was different. Some lasted a couple of hours, others lasted a couple of days. It depended on what God wanted for the child. In the Sacred Dream, the child heard things they had not heard before. This was the voice of God. The child also saw things that did not exist. This is what God wanted the child to see. It was the job of the Healer/Priest to help the child interpret the meaning of the Sacred Dream given by God. It was important for each member of the village to be spiritually strong and pass through the rite of passage.

If the child objected to the profession chosen by God in the Sacred Dream, the child's spirit stayed in heaven and the body died. This is why white people object to the Chumash Religion and make sure that it is labeled felony child endangerment. There is a racist misperception that the Chumash people killed their own children. In traditional times, the children were the future of the community and were considered precious. Did children actually die? Children who were born with severe birth defects that made it impossible for them to be productive did not survive the rite of passage. This amounted to very few children.

Inbreeding was a serious concern in traditional times. The villages were small, with about 100 people. When first cousins marry, there is a real risk of serious birth defects in the children. My teacher told me the Chumash people would breed with "anyone who came over the mountain." In other words, they sought new genetic material from people from distant places. This is why Cabrillo and other explorers found Chumash women interested in breeding with them.

The US Constitution guarantees religious freedom for everyone. The Chumash Religion is still considered illegal. It may be many years before white people can overcome their racism and allow the Chumash Religion to return to California.

10.2. Second Sacred Dream

The second Sacred Dream occurred when a couple wanted to marry. The elders of the village had to agree to the marriage. This was to prevent inbreeding and to maintain the balance of the village. The Healer/Priest made preparation of Momoy for them to ingest that differed from the first preparation. This preparation was weaker and less of a challenge. Both people had already gone through the rite of passage and had earned their places in the village.

In the second Sacred Dream, God taught each person how to be a good spouse. The man was told to never cheat on his wife, always be faithful and honest with her. The woman was taught not to scream at her husband and to be kind to him. When both agreed to God's teaching, their spirits returned to their bodies. Momoy does not cause sexual stimulation.

10.3. Third Sacred Dream

The third Sacred Dream occurred when a couple had been given permission to have a baby. A birth could only occur when an elder died and made a place for the child. This is how the balance was maintained in the village. In this Sacred Dream, the husband and wife were taught how to raise a child, to teach the child to be productive, and not make excuses for the child. When the couple agreed to God's teaching, their spirits returned to their bodies. They were then given permission to have vaginal sex. Prior to this, other forms of sex that did not result in pregnancy were allowed.

When the child was born, the entire village took part in raising the child. Each child was considered precious and essential to the survival of the village. Even children that had been born with severe birth defects were cared for. Some of these children learned to be productive in the village and survived the rite of passage. Each village then had the burden of deciding if that person with a severe birth defect would be allowed to marry and have a child.

10.4. Fourth Sacred Dream

The fourth Sacred Dream occurred when it was time for someone to die. Each person got to die with dignity, to choose the time and place of their death. Of course, this was done in consultation with the Healer/Priest. The fourth sacred dream involved a different preparation of Momoy administered in a different way. In this Sacred Dream, the spirit went to God, who welcomed the spirit and put the spirit on the path to heaven.

10.5. Momoy Dose

The dose of Momoy is critical to the Sacred Dream; too much will cause respiratory depression, too little will result in no dream [14, 30]. My teacher taught me that for most teenage boys, the dose is about 40 seeds, depending on how much they weigh. The dose for girls is less, about 20 - 30 seeds, depending on the weight of the girl. The seeds must be carefully ground in a stone mortar with a stone pestle. If the seeds are not ground, scopolamine will not be released after ingestion. The seeds will pass through the guts and will not produce a Sacred Dream.

It is important to fast for 12 h before starting the sacred dream. I have realized that the flowers are easier to work with and easier to get the correct dose with. The flowers are doorways to the future since they produce seeds that create the next generation. I cut the flowers into quarters lengthwise and start with a quarter of a flower. The person chews the quarter flower and swallows. After 30 min, if the person experiences no effects, such as dry mouth, I administer another quarter or eighth of a flower and wait 30 min. This continues until the person experiences a dry mouth or up to the terminal dose. I do not administer more than three-quarters of a flower for someone under 140 lbs (63.5 kg) or an entire flower for someone over 140 lbs. When the person has a dry mouth, that is usually the sign that the proper dose has been given. The half-life of scopolamine is 9.5 h. Most of the scopolamine is still in the body 30 min after administration.

The symptoms that appear are dry mouth that can be very uncomfortable, decreased visual acuity, visual hallucinations, auditory hallucinations, increased perception of colors, sense of hearing, taste and smell. Sexual stimulation does not occur. Higher doses are not recommended since hyperthermia, respiratory depression and compromised visual acuity can result. The visual hallucinations can be interpreted as something God wants the person to see. The auditory hallucinations can be interpreted to be the voice of God or something God wants the person to hear. Sometimes an animal appears in the Sacred Dream and is the Dream Guide for the person. The Healer/Priest helps the person interpret the Sacred Dream. Unfortunately, white people who abuse Momoy do not understand this. Sometimes they panic, which can result in accidents and self-harm.

The levels of scopolamine in the seeds of *D. stramonium*, a cousin of *D. wrightii*, are about 0.4 ug/mg of atropine and 0.1 ug/mg of scopolamine in the seeds [31]. The CDC reports 0.1 mg of atropine (hyoscyamine) and 0.05 mg of scopolamine per seed [32]. This may be a typographical error. Perhaps the actual levels are 0.1 ug of atropine and 0.05 ug of scopolamine per seed. Another report found 2.7 ug/mg of atropine in the seeds and 0.7 ug/mg of scopolamine in the seeds [33]. The dried flowers contain 0.3 ug/mg of hyoscyamine and 0.07 ug/mg of scopolamine [31]. Each flower weighs about 4 g when fresh or about 0.4 g when dried. Each flower contains about 1.2 mg of hyoscyamine and 280 ug of scopolamine. The usual adult intravenous dosage of scopolamine in perioperative sedation is 320-650 ug, as discussed in Drug Facts and Comparisons. Similarly, hyoscyamine is used clinically in intravenous doses of 5ug/kg body weight. This is 400 ug in an 80 kg adult.

The oral bioavailability of scopolamine is variable in terms of penetration across the gut and across the blood-brain barrier. Gut penetration results in 11-48% of oral scopolamine appearing in the blood [34]. There is a 4 fold difference in oral bioavailability between people. This makes dosing with scopolamine difficult and potentially dangerous. Atropine has 25% oral bioavailability. Most people, about 85%, have rapid penetration of scopolamine into the brain and experience symptoms within 20 min [30]. However, about 1 out of 6 people has a slow penetration of scopolamine into the brain. Some of these people can require up to 12 hours before scopolamine penetrates into the brain and symptoms occur. It is very easy to for these people to overdose with Momoy. That is why no more than three-quarters of a flower for people under 63.5 kg or one flower for people over 63.5 kg should be administered.

Assuming 50% bioavailability for scopolamine and 25% bioavailability for atropine as discussed in Drug Facts and Comparisons, the oral dose from one flower delivers 300 ug of hyoscyamine and 140 ug of scopolamine to the blood, or 440 ug total. This is similar to the normal clinical intravenous doses of atropine and scopolamine. Of course, these drugs have similar, probably additive, interactions with brain muscarinic receptors.

10.6. Vision Quests

The Healer/Priests, and other people went on vision quests as needed. This involved going alone into the wilderness, fasting, and praying. Sometimes the person chose to spend the night on top of a ridge or mountain. The person chose the place to sleep. A Sacred Dream would come that provided some direction or answers to questions. Vision quests were just as important as Sacred Dreams associated with Momoy.

10.7. Fire Tending

When a person was old enough, they passed through the fire tending vigil. This involved spending the night alone while praying and keeping a small fire burning all night long. This ritual showed the community the person was ready to take on the responsibility of taking care of the village and could undergo hardships to ensure the comfort of others.

11. CARLOS CASTANEDA

My teacher's grandparents taught Carlos Castaneda. They were all Chumash Healer/Priests who returned to California from exile in Mexico. They came from 4 different places in Mexico, Ignacio Alvarez, Refugio Alvarez, Geronimo Garcia and Cecilia Garcia (the grandmother). One of the grandparents had lived in Hermosillo and was a Healer/Priest to the Yaqui people. They decided to teach

Castaneda since he was Latino and was studying to become an Anthropologist. They hoped that being Latino meant he would not lie to them. They hoped his credentials in Anthropology would help white people listen to what he might say about the Chumash teachings.

Castaneda was not a good student and frequently did not show up when he was supposed to. He lied to his teachers, friends and the public that read his books. He did not have the courage to take Momoy. Instead he used LSD and peyote. He wrote some very popular books that he never proved to be factual. He claimed to have been taught by the Yaqui people when he was actually taught by the Chumash people. He did nothing to help the Chumash Religion or his teachers.

12. PSYCHEDELIC AS A REPLACEMENT FOR SACRED MEDICINES

Many Sacred Medicines used in Sacred Dreams are also used as psychedelic agents, such as peyote, psilocybe mushrooms and ayahuasca. Ayahuasca can be made from *Psychotria viridis* and *Banisteriopsis caapi,* as has been retold in many accounts. In the opinion of the author, psychedelic means that in addition to causing visual hallucinations, they are sexual stimulants, similar to LSD. The Healer/Priests who use these Sacred Medicines must carefully teach their students how to be open to Sacred Dreams and not sexual stimulation. However, it is the author's perception that among the psychedelic drug community, sexual stimulation is a desirable aspect of these medicines. Perhaps psychedelic drugs are used to treat depression and other conditions partly because they are sexual stimulants. Fortunately, some people who use psychedelic drugs report having sacred experiences. For this reason, some people call these medicines entheogens. In fact, the author worked with Alexander Shulgin, who synthesized many entheogens, even though he did not believe in God [35]. It is the experience of the author that Scientists who work with entheogens rarely mention God. I have been told that mentioning God is not objective.

In the Amazon jungle, both ayahuasca and *Brugmansia* are found. There are several species of *Brugmansia* in the Amazon, such as *B. insignis*, *B. versicolor* and others. *B. suaveolens* is reported to be extinct in the Amazon, but is grown in gardens around the world. *Brugmansia* species are all used as sacred medicines, contain scopolamine and hyoscyamine [36]. In many areas of the Amazon, *Brugmansia* is used rather than ayahuasca. There are reports in the press and popular magazines that *Brugmansia* causes violent convulsions, foaming of the mouth and stupor for many hours. It is unlikely that an Amazonian Indian mother would want her child to go through an experience like that. It is likely the popular reports are exaggerated. Scopolamine causes dry mouth and is unlikely to cause foaming of the mouth.

Many people in the psychedelic community insist that ayahuasca is safe and no one has ever died from ayahuasca. This is not true. There are several reports of people who have died from vomiting or reactivation of psychosis caused by ayahuasca [37 - 42]. Vomiting causes death by aspiration and rupture of the esophagus.

Many people in the psychedelic community self-treat their depression or bipolar disorder with psychedelic agents. This is rarely effective and frequently does more harm than good. Perhaps these agents are being used as escape mechanisms to escape from depression or bipolar disorder. The most effective treatment for depression or bipolar disorder is regular, daily exercise, such as running [43].

13. PICTOGRAPHS

The Chumash pictographs are world famous (Fig. **2**). They were created in the past by Healer/Priests to aid in healing and predicting the future [44]. When a patient with a very difficult disease presented for healing, the Healer/Priest would pray so that God could teach the correct treatment. When this was not enough, the Healer/Priest would use Momoy to induce a Sacred Dream. The spirit of the Healer/Priest went to God for direct instruction. Sometimes the Healer/Priest experienced a very vivid Sacred Dream that resulted in a trance difficult for others to interpret, such as excitation, dancing and speaking unintelligibly.

Very beautiful pictographs were painted in a fertility site called Pleito. Gonorrhea brought by the Spanish made fertility a difficult issue to cure. These pictographs depict the penis, vagina, uterus and other symbols meant to help the couple with their fertility.

CONCLUSIONS

Each of us has the potential for spirituality. If we choose, we could use this spirituality to enhance our lives and help motivate us to live in balance. Spirituality is a choice that we can make. It is important to respect the spirituality of others and not take away religious freedom for the sake of racism or abuse.

REFERENCES

[1]   Janssen-Niemeijer AJ, Visse M, Van Leeuwen R, Leget C, Cusveller BS. The role of spirituality in lifestyle changing among patients with chronic cardiovascular diseases: A literature review of qualitative studies. J Relig Health 2017; 56(4): 1460-77.
[http://dx.doi.org/10.1007/s10943-017-0384-2] [PMID: 28349298]

[2]   El Magboub A, Garcia C, Adams JD. A revival of primary healing hypotheses: A comparison of traditional healing approaches of Arabs and American Indians. Tang Int J Genuine Traditional Med 2012; 2(1): 1-14.

[http://dx.doi.org/10.5667/tang.2011.0025]

[3]   Renugadevi R. Environmental ethics in the Hindu Vedas and Puranas in India. African J History Culture 2012; 4(1): 1-3.
      [http://dx.doi.org/10.5897/AJHC11.042]

[4]   Aich TK. Buddha philosophy and western psychology. Indian J Psychiatry 2013; 55 (Suppl. 2): S165-70.
      [http://dx.doi.org/10.4103/0019-5545.105517] [PMID: 23858249]

[5]   Wallace BA, Shapiro SL. Mental balance and well-being: building bridges between Buddhism and Western psychology. Am Psychol 2006; 61(7): 690-701.
      [http://dx.doi.org/10.1037/0003-066X.61.7.690] [PMID: 17032069]

[6]   Levey J, Levey M. Living in Balance. A Mindful Guide for Thriving in a Complex World. New York: Divine Arts 2014.

[7]   Tucker M, Berthrong J. Confucianism and Ecology Volume. Boston: Center for the Study of World Religions 1998.

[8]   Adams JD, Garcia C, Lien EJ. A comparison of Chinese and Chumash Medicine. ECAM 2008.
      [http://dx.doi.org/10.1093/ecam/nem188]

[9]   Adams JD. DNA, Nuclear Cell Signaling and Neurodegeneration. In: Adams JD, Parker K, Eds. Extracellular and intracellular signaling. London: Royal Society of Chemistry 2011; pp. 175-87.
      [http://dx.doi.org/10.1039/9781849733434-00175]

[10] Adams JD, Lien EJ. The Traditional and Scientific Bases for Traditional Chinese Medicine: Communication between Traditional Practitioners, Physicians and Scientists.Traditional Chinese medicine – scientific basis for its use. London: Royal Society of Chemistry 2013; pp. 1-10.
      [http://dx.doi.org/10.1039/9781849737852-00001]

[11] Lien EJ, Lien LL, Adams JD. Structure Activity Relationship Analysis of Plant Derived Compounds.Traditional Chinese medicine – scientific basis for its use. London: Royal Society of Chemistry 2013; pp. 11-6.
      [http://dx.doi.org/10.1039/9781849737852-00011]

[12] Rush D. Vodun in Coastal Benin: Unfinished, Open-Ended, Global (Critical Investigations of the African Diaspora). Nashville: Vanderbilt University Press 2013.

[13] Davis EW. The ethnobiology of the Haitian zombi. J Ethnopharmacol 1983; 9(1): 85-104.
      [http://dx.doi.org/10.1016/0378-8741(83)90029-6] [PMID: 6668953]

[14] Adams J, Wong M, Villasenor E. Healing with medicinal plants of the west – cultural and scientific basis for their use fourth edition. La Crescenta: Abedus Press 2020.

[15] Adams JD, Garcia C. The spiritual sense, prayer and traditional American Indian healing. TANG Int J Genuine Traditional Med 2012; 2(1): 1-6.
      [http://dx.doi.org/10.5667/tang.2011.0012]

[16] Blackburn T. December's Child a Book of Chumash Oral Narratives. Berkeley: University of California Press 1975.

[17] Laird C. Encounter with an Angry God: Recollections of My Life with John Peabody Harrington Banning. Malki Museum Press 1975.

[18] Hudson T, Underhay E. Crystals in the Sky: An Intellectual Odyssey Involving Chumash Astronomy, Cosmology and Rock Art. Santa Barbara: Ballena Press 1978.

[19] Hudson T, Blackburn T, Curletti R, Timbrook J, Eds. The Eye of the Flute: Chumash Traditional History and Ritual as Told by Fernando Librado Kitsepawit to John P. Harrington. Illustrated by Campbell Grant. Santa Barbara: Santa Barbara Museum of Natural History, Santa Barbara Bicentennial Historical Series 1977.

[20]   Kramer W. Juan Rodriguez Cabrillo a Voyage of Rediscovery. San Diego: Maritime Museum of San Diego 2019.

[21]   [Desert Sun]: "Berkeley — A University of California anthropologist believes he has found the grave marker of Juan Rodriguez Cabrillo, the Spanish "discoverer of California." 1972.

[22]   Adams J, Phipps T. Los Angeles Indian Labor Practices after the Civil War. J West 2018; 57: 60-71.

[23]   Adams J, Phipps T. Los Angeles Area Indian Land Ownership After the Civil War. J West 2018; 57: 7-13.

[24]   Trafzer C, Hyer J. Exterminate Them: Written Accounts of Murder, Rape and Enslavement of Native Americans During the California Gold Rush. An Arbor: University of Michigan Press. 1999.

[25]   Madley B. An American Genocide the United States and the California Indian Catastrophe. New Haven: Yale University Press 2016.

[26]   Smith S. Freedom's Frontier California and The Struggle Over Unfree Labor, Emancipation, and Reconstruction. Chapel Hill: University of North Carolina Press 2013.

[27]   Lindsay B. Murder State California's Native American Genocide 1846-1873. Lincoln: University of Nebraska Press 2012.
[http://dx.doi.org/10.2307/j.ctt1d9nqs3]

[28]   Carrico R. Strangers in a stolen land Indians of San Diego County from prehistory to the new deal. San Diego: Sunbelt Publications 2008.

[29]   Heizer R. The destruction of California Indians. Lincoln: University of Nebraska Press 1993.

[30]   Adams J, Garcia C. The advantages of traditional Chumash healing. eCAM 2005; 2(1): 19-23.
[http://dx.doi.org/10.1093/ecam/neh072]

[31]   Miraldi E, Masti A, Ferri S, Barni Comparini I. Distribution of hyoscyamine and scopolamine in Datura stramonium. Fitoterapia 2001; 72(6): 644-8.
[http://dx.doi.org/10.1016/S0367-326X(01)00291-X] [PMID: 11543961]

[32]   Centers for disease control and prevention. Leads from the morbidity and mortality weekly report: Jimson weed poisoning Texas, New York and California 1994. J Am Med Assoc 1995; 273: 532-3.
[http://dx.doi.org/10.1001/jama.1995.03520310026022]

[33]   Dugan GM, Gumbmann MR, Friedman M. Toxicological evaluation of jimson weed (Datura stramonium) seed. Food Chem Toxicol 1989; 27(8): 501-10.
[http://dx.doi.org/10.1016/0278-6915(89)90045-8] [PMID: 2792973]

[34]   Putcha L, Cintrón NM, Tsui J, Vanderploeg JM, Kramer WG. Pharmacokinetics and oral bioavailability of scopolamine in normal subjects. Pharm Res 1989; 6(6): 481-5.
[http://dx.doi.org/10.1023/A:1015916423156] [PMID: 2762223]

[35]   Shulgin A, Shulgin A. PIKHAL a Chemical Love Story. Berkeley: Transform Press 1991.

[36]   Evans W, Lampard J. Alkaloids of Datura suaveolens. Phytochemistry 1972; 11(11): 3293-8.
[http://dx.doi.org/10.1016/S0031-9422(00)86392-X]

[37]   Parkin Daniels J. Colombia's Ayahuasca Ceremonies in Spotlight after Tourist's Drug Death. The Guardian 2018.

[38]   Macdonald H. How an ayahuasca retreat claimed the life of a 24yo Kiwi tourist in the Amazon. https://www.abc.net.au/triplej/programs/hack/how-ayahuasca-retreat-claimed-the-life-of-a--4yo-kiwi-tourist/83503382017.

[39]   Ray K. No charges filed after death at ayahuasca church https://www.ajc.com/news/national/charges-filed-after-death-ayahuasca-church/N49bd39evkLCqXV8PXeKlM/2018.

[40]   Sklerov J, Levine B, Moore KA, King T, Fowler D. A fatal intoxication following the ingestion of 5-methoxy-N,N-dimethyltryptamine in an ayahuasca preparation. J Anal Toxicol 2005; 29(8): 838-41.

[http://dx.doi.org/10.1093/jat/29.8.838] [PMID: 16356341]

[41]   McVeigh T. "British backpacker dies after taking hallucinogenic brew in Colombia". The Observer 2014.

[42]   Wiltshire PE, Hawksworth DL, Edwards KJ. Light microscopy can reveal the consumption of a mixture of psychotropic plant and fungal material in suspicious death. J Forensic Leg Med 2015; 34: 73-80.
[http://dx.doi.org/10.1016/j.jflm.2015.05.010] [PMID: 26165663]

[43]   Johnsgard K. The exercise prescription for depression and anxiety. Cambridge: Da Capo Press 1989.

[44]   Adams J, Garcia C. Spirit, mind and body in Chumash healing. eCAM 2005; 1-5.
[http://dx.doi.org/10.1093/ecam/neh130]

CHAPTER 3

The Family and Balance

Abstract: Balance in the family depends on having positive attitudes, good communication and the ability to make decisions together. Families must be able to adapt to challenges such as the end of life, serious diseases, depression, mental disorders, and poor health decisions such as obesity. Child abuse can tear families apart. More approaches to the treatment of adults who are child abusers are needed.

1. INTRODUCTION

Childhood development, mental and physical health are influenced by the family [1]. It is important for the family to provide a supportive, positive and stable environment for the child to develop. This is a challenge for most families, given the economic and political changes that are occurring in the world today. Of course, the mental and physical well-being of the parents is supported by good family health as well.

The life balance model [2] can be modified to define family balance. Family balance is a satisfying pattern of daily activity that is healthful, meaningful and sustainable to a family within the life circumstances of the family. Everyday family activities should: be safe and enhance biological health; involve rewarding and self-affirming relationships; help family members feel engaged, challenged and competent; create a family identity. This model has been tested and validated in terms of individual life balance [2] and could be tested as a model of family balance.

Balance is important in family health and is defined as balancing time spent at work, together with the family, during social activities and taking care of oneself [1]. Families must prioritize the family and devote time together such as in the morning, evening, weekends and on vacation. This helps families have shared visions of future goals and supportive communication.

Awareness and reflection are mediators of family health [1]. Each member should be aware of the needs of other members and the problems created by the actions of others. Bad behavior such as lying and stealing should not be tolerated and not excused.Positive reflection and supportive communication can help modify behavior and lead to improved family health. Rewarding good behavior and good performance reinforces this behavior.

The family needs to adjust, adapt and change as the family situation changes [1]. This includes changes in employment, births, deaths and other changes. Families have identities based on shared experiences, beliefs, values and preferences. This identity may change as the family matures together and shares new experiences.

Each family experiences trying times, such as loss of employment, chronic illness, or senility [1]. Families that adapt to these challenges have better family health. It is during trying times that the bad behavior of one member can damage the family. This bad behavior must be met with positive reflection and supportive communication.

Kindness, repentance and forgiveness are critical to individual and family health [3, 4]. Of course, family members love each other, but are they kind to each other? Kindness and love are very different qualities to some people. It is common for an abusive parent to tell the child, "I love you. But I have to teach you a lesson. I am doing this for your own good." Kindness means to be generous and considerate without expecting a reward. Repentance involves an apology, making changes to ensure the mistake does not happen again and making restitution to compensate for the damage done. Forgiveness means accepting repentance without retaliation.

2. CONSEQUENCES OF FAMILY LIFE

Adults make sacrifices for their families [5]. Women, especially, find it hard to advance their careers while being mothers. With housing prices and the cost of living to increase, it is required for both partners in a marriage to work in order to buy a house and live as a family. On the other hand, working can make it more difficult to be a parent, especially for women. About 28% of working parents had to decrease work hours or take significant time off to take care of their families. About 15% of parents had to quit work to take care of their families. However, nearly 90% of parents who experienced career interruptions did not regret these experiences.

3. CARING FOR FAMILY MEMBERS AT THE END OF LIFE

Caring for a mother, father or other family members at the end of life is very challenging [6]. As the cost of long-term health care for these patients becomes prohibitive for most families, a family member is usually assigned to care for the dying family member. Frequently, the patient will display bad behavior such as abusive language and uncooperative behavior. It is important not to make excuses for this behavior. The family must support the person who has been assigned to provide health care. Sometimes, temporary nursing care is purchased to help during trying times. It is best for the family and the patient when the family remains a cohesive unit.

The most difficult decision for many families is physician-assisted death. Especially for families of patients suffering from Alzheimer's disease, the monthly assisted living cost is exorbitant and is not covered by health insurance. As discussed in the spirituality chapter, during traditional times, the Chumash Indians of California allowed these patients to decide when and where to end their lives. In this way, they died with dignity and were not a burden to their families. Physician-assisted death is not illegal in 10 states in the US [7]. Patients must be suffering from a terminal illness with no more than 6 months to live. This precludes patients suffering from Alzheimer's disease. So far, physician assisted death is used by several hundred patients yearly in the US.

Alzheimer's disease has become a major burden for many families since medicine can keep people alive long enough to develop the disease. Even after being diagnosed with Alzheimer's disease, it is common for patients to live another 7 years or more. The cause of Alzheimer's disease is not known. For many years, the dogma was that amyloid caused the disease. This dogma was supported by many publications. However, drugs that decrease brain amyloid plaques do not ameliorate Alzheimer's disease [8]. It is obvious that the disease is caused by other mechanisms, such as a leaky blood-brain barrier [9].

Cancer is another severe challenge for families. Families must not panic and remember that cancer is no longer a death sentence. Up to 70% or more cancer patients survive most cancers. Family members can become caregivers to cancer patients, including driving patients to doctor's appointments, chemotherapy and surgery visits, helping patients understand the disease and its treatments, helping patients with the side effects of chemotherapy, and more [10]. A critical therapy the family can provide is to cheer up the patient and help them avoid depression. The family should discuss "what if" scenarios with the patient so they are prepared for what might happen. The patient should also appoint one family member to help make do not resuscitate or other end-of-life decisions for the patient if necessary.

4. CARING FOR DEPRESSED FAMILY MEMBERS

Depression is a disorder that affects 3% of people and costs $210 billion every year in the US. This disorder is characterized by a depressed mood that is present most of the time, low self-esteem, loss of interest, and pain. About 4% of patients commit suicide and many more attempt suicide. The cause of depression is not known. Antidepressant drugs are available and are associated with remission in about half of patients. However, relapses and failed therapy are common. Many studies have found little or no effect of antidepressant medicines compared to placebo [11]. These drugs are all toxic and must be used for the rest of the patient's life. Many patients and their families choose not to use these drugs. Loving caregivers in the family are important for depressed patients. Patients who thought their caregivers loved them were more than 40% less likely to have suicidal ideation [4].

The most effective treatment for depression, bipolar disorder and anxiety is daily aerobic exercise, such as running, walking, swimming and bicycling [12]. Exercise should be sustained and last about an hour. About 80% effort is best such that the patient does not become over-exerted. This allows the exercise to occur daily. The patient must perform an hour of exercise daily for the remainder of their life. Fortunately, the human body is designed to perform daily exercise. The body and mind benefit from daily exercise.

The family of depressed, bipolar and anxiety patients can help motivate the patient to exercise, such as by accompanying the patient on walks, runs or bicycle rides. Positive reinforcement and supportive communication will help the patient and the family.

Ketamine is the drug of choice for the prevention of suicide [13]. This drug blocks N-methyl-D-aspartate receptors and abolishes suicidal thoughts within minutes after injection. Ketamine is also a pain reliever that has been used as an anesthetic [14]. This drug is used as a last resort in patients at extreme risk and is not used as a daily treatment.

5. CARING FOR MENTALLY ILL FAMILY MEMBERS

Schizophrenia, schizoaffective disorder, and delusional disorders are major challenges for the family. Many families are unable to help or even live with patients affected by these disorders. Many of these patients end up homeless and live on the streets. These disorders can be characterized by delusions, psychosis, paranoia, disorganized thinking, abnormal motor behavior, lack of motivation, poverty of speech, and other symptoms. The causes of these disorders are not known.

Many drugs are available to treat these mental disorders. Most of the antipsychotic agents are dopamine receptor 2 antagonists. This suggests that dopamine is somehow involved in causing or exacerbating psychosis. All of these drugs are toxic. They can cause extrapyramidal side effects in 50% of patients. This involves parkinsonism, tremor, dystonia and akathisia. These symptoms usually subside once the drug is stopped. More serious and potentially irreversible side effects of these drugs include tardive dyskinesia, neuroleptic malignant disorder and shortened life span [15, 16].

Family members should be careful not to take sides for or against the wishes of the mentally ill patient. It is best for the family to discuss the needed therapy for the patient and to be united in their decision. The patient rarely goes into therapy voluntarily. Coercion is routinely used to force the patient into therapy [17]. Several important concerns must be addressed, including the safety of family members and health care workers when dealing with potentially violent patients. The police frequently become involved when the behavior of the patient becomes a threat to the community. The patient is then coerced into involuntary therapy which can involve psychotherapy, family therapy, hospitalization, high-security hospitalization or incarceration. Family members may feel coerced by this process and express feelings that: it was necessary but terrible; the family could not stay connected with the patient; the patient may have been harmed; the drug therapy may be harmful. The family needs to communicate with health care professionals to be convinced that the therapy is appropriate and the correct decision for the patient. Health care professionals should be sensitive to the needs of the family and help them with this difficult decision.

Patients usually remain on antipsychotic medication for the rest of their lives. However, there are reports of patients recovering and realizing that their delusions are actually just delusions. The efficacy of antipsychotic drugs is poor, except for clozapine which, according to meta-analysis, is the only antipsychotic that is effective in treatment-resistant psychosis [18].

6. CHILD ABUSE

Perhaps the ugliest aspect of family life is the potential for child abuse (Table **1**). Parents, teachers and other adults that have authority over children may abuse children sexually, physically, emotionally or by neglect. The stories of child abuse are difficult to hear, especially stories of parents selling their children into sexual slavery.

Table 1. Child abuse characteristics adapted from https://www.childhelp.org/child-abuse/.

Type of Abuse	Characteristics	Symptoms in the Child	Prevalence
Sexual abuse of boys and girls	Adults or older children coerce children to participate in sexual activities	Difficulty sitting or walking, bowel problems, sexually transmitted diseases, can result in depression, withdrawal, sleep disturbances	21% of US adults report being physically abused as a child
Physical abuse	Adults or older children intentionally injure a child	Unexplained injuries including broken bones, can result in aggression, nightmares and self-destructive behavior	28% of US adults report being sexually abused as a child
Emotional abuse	Adults or older children harm the mental or social development of a child such as by repeated berating	Developmental delays, speech disorders, obesity, can result in learning disability, antisocial behavior	11% of US adults report being emotionally abused as a child
Neglect abuse	Adults do not provide the care needed by the child by inadequate supervision, emotional, medical or educational neglect	Low body weight, untreated medical problems, hygiene problems, can result in truancy, feelings of inadequacy, depression	60% of child abuse victims are neglected

It is important to understand that child abuse involves adults abusing the child and adults ignoring the problem [19]. For instance, if a mother abuses her daughter physically and emotionally, the father must ignore the problem and allow the abuse to occur. If a teacher abuses a student, the parents are involved in the problem since they allow the problem to persist by ignoring the problem. Parents must be very careful about allowing any adult to have authority over their children. Parents must be involved or supervise the activities of their children as much as possible. It is possible that with parent, religious leader or healthcare professional intervention, the child abuse can be stopped.

The sad reality is that adults who abuse children frequently do not stop and can be serial child abusers. Sometimes, the only way to stop child abuse by a parent is to permanently separate the parent from the child, such as by divorce or putting the child into foster care. Adults who abuse children that are not their own may continue to abuse other children even after being arrested and jailed. Half of all children who have been abused will be abused again [19].

The consequences of being an abused child are major [20]. When the child becomes an adult, depression, chronic pain, memory problems, cognitive difficulties and other problems can interfere with life and make a living a normal life impossible [21]. Nightmares and flashbacks of the abuse are common and are psychologically devastating. Another consequence is that child abuse usually involves only one child. Other children in the family may be completely unaware of the abuse of a sibling and may not believe that abuse has occurred. This disbelief can tear siblings apart and destroy the family.

7. CARING FOR A CHILD WITH CEREBRAL PALSY

Disabled children, such as children born with cerebral palsy, have long-term impacts on the family [22]. The parents must adjust their careers to take care of the child and must find the resources they need for this care. Parents must also become educated about the disability and how to care for the child.

Cerebral palsy is caused by brain damage in the fetus or at birth. It is the most common motor disability in children affecting 1 in 323. Children born by *in vitro* fertilization are more commonly affected by cerebral palsy. The Centers for Disease Control write that with the proper support and services people affected by cerebral palsy can be active members of the community.

It falls to the family to find and provide the support and services the patient needs. This produces significant stress in the family. About one-third of parents caring for cerebral palsy patients require healthcare professional assistance [22]. The parents must monitor the motor behavior of their children and help them reach the milestones required for good development. However, the behavioral problems of their children are the most difficult to deal with. A good functioning family that supports each other with positive attitudes is essential to deal with these behavioral problems. Providing respite for the parents can also help. This may involve bringing in a home healthcare nurse temporarily.

8. CARING FOR AN OBESE CHILD

Childhood obesity became a problem in the 1980s when adult obesity became a problem [23]. The health consequences of obesity are discussed in the lifestyle chapter. Children learn eating habits from their parents. When the parents are obese, the children may not be discouraged from becoming obese. Children also learn exercise habits from their parent's examples. If the parents find exercise unnecessary, the children may not feel encouraged to exercise. One approach to the obesity problem is to encourage parents to get rid of excess weight, and by example, encourage the children to do the same [24]. School-based obesity programs have been shown in several studies to be effective and can involve school nurses [25]. Children are encouraged to eat vegetables and fruits, decrease recreational video games and television time, enjoy 1 hour of physical activity daily and avoid sugary drinks. These programs result in less obesity and increased health measures in children. A possible result of school-based obesity programs is that children set the example for adults in the family.

CONCLUSIONS

In order for people to thrive, it is best to have a supportive, positive family environment. Healthcare providers can ask questions about the family to find out what the family environment is like. They can also help with education to help the family understand the importance of the family in therapy for a sick patient. Healthcare providers must not avoid the responsibility of reporting possible child abuse. This is frequently the only hope for victims of child abuse.

REFERENCES

[1]   Smith SL, DeGrace B, Ciro C, *et al.* Exploring families' experiences of health: contributions to a model of family health. Psychol Health Med 2017; 22(10): 1239-47.
       [http://dx.doi.org/10.1080/13548506.2017.1319069] [PMID: 28425318]

[2]   Matuska K. Validity Evidence of a Model and Measure of Life Balance. OTJR (Thorofare, NJ) 2012; 32(1): 229-37.
       [http://dx.doi.org/10.3928/15394492-20110610-02]

[3]   Clabby JF. Forgiveness: Moving on *can* be healthy. Int J Psychiatry Med 2020; 55(2): 123-30.
       [http://dx.doi.org/10.1177/0091217419885468] [PMID: 31735110]

[4]   Susukida R, Wilcox HC, Mendelson T. The association of lifetime suicidal ideation with perceived parental love and family structure in childhood in a nationally representative adult sample. Psychiatry Res 2016; 237: 246-51.
       [http://dx.doi.org/10.1016/j.psychres.2016.01.033] [PMID: 26803361]

[5]   Pew Research Center. On pay Gap, Millennial Women Near Parity – For Now Despite Gains Many Roadblocks Ahead. Washington, D.C.: Pew Research Center 2013.

[6]   Anderson EW, White KM. "This is what family does": The family experience of caring for serious illness. Am J Hospice Palliative Med 2018; 35(2): 348-54.
       [http://dx.doi.org/10.1177/1049909117709251] [PMID: 28662594]

[7]   https://www.cnn.com/2014/11/26/us/physician-assisted-suicide-fast-facts/index.html

[8]   Adams J. The treatment of brain inflammation in alzheimer's disease. Can traditional medicines help? Frontiers Clin Drug Res Alzheimer Disorders 2016; 6: 1-19.

[9]   Adams JD Jr. Alzheimer's disease, ceramide, visfatin and NAD. CNS Neurol Disord Drug Targets 2008; 7(6): 492-8.
       [http://dx.doi.org/10.2174/187152708787122969] [PMID: 19128206]

[10]   Dionne-Odom JN, Ejem D, Wells R, *et al.* How family caregivers of persons with advanced cancer assist with upstream healthcare decision-making: A qualitative study. PLoS One 2019; 14(3): e0212967.
       [http://dx.doi.org/10.1371/journal.pone.0212967] [PMID: 30865681]

[11]   Khan A, Brown WA. Antidepressants *versus* placebo in major depression: an overview. World Psychiatry 2015; 14(3): 294-300.
       [http://dx.doi.org/10.1002/wps.20241] [PMID: 26407778]

[12]   Johnsgard KW. The Exercise Prescription for Depression and Anxiety. New York: Plenum Press 1989.

[13]   Matveychuk D, Thomas RK, Swainson J, *et al.* Ketamine as an antidepressant: overview of its mechanisms of action and potential predictive biomarkers. Ther Adv Psychopharmacol 2020; 10: 2045125320916657.
[http://dx.doi.org/10.1177/2045125320916657] [PMID: 32440333]

[14]   Adams JD Jr, Baillie TA, Trevor AJ, Castagnoli N Jr. Studies on the biotransformation of ketamine. 1-Identification of metabolites produced *in vitro* from rat liver microsomal preparations. Biomed Mass Spectrom 1981; 8(11): 527-38.
[http://dx.doi.org/10.1002/bms.1200081103] [PMID: 7317567]

[15]   Ballon JS, Pajvani U, Freyberg Z, Leibel RL, Lieberman JA. Molecular pathophysiology of metabolic effects of antipsychotic medications. Trends Endocrinol Metab 2014; 25(11): 593-600.
[http://dx.doi.org/10.1016/j.tem.2014.07.004] [PMID: 25190097]

[16]   Adams J. Tardive dyskinesia and dopamine oxidation, cumulative effects. J Multidisc Sci J 2019; 2: 138-41.
[http://dx.doi.org/10.3390/j2020011]

[17]   Norvoll R, Hem MH, Lindemann H. Family Members' Existential and Moral Dilemmas With Coercion in Mental Healthcare. Qual Health Res 2018; 28(6): 900-15.journals.sagepub.com/home/qhr
[http://dx.doi.org/10.1177/1049732317750120] [PMID: 29310541]

[18]   Lally J, MacCabe JH. Antipsychotic medication in schizophrenia: a review. Br Med Bull 2015; 114(1): 169-79.
[http://dx.doi.org/10.1093/bmb/ldv017] [PMID: 25957394]

[19]   McDonald KC. Child abuse: approach and management. Am Fam Physician 2007; 75(2): 221-8.
[PMID: 17263217]

[20]   Mark CA, Poltavski DV, Petros T, King A. Differential executive functioning in young adulthood as a function of experienced child abuse. Int J Psychophysiol 2019; 135: 126-35.
[http://dx.doi.org/10.1016/j.ijpsycho.2018.12.004] [PMID: 30552916]

[21]   Alhalal E, Ford-Gilboe M, Wong C, AlBuhairan F. Factors mediating the impacts of child abuse and intimate partner violence on chronic pain: a cross-sectional study. BMC Womens Health 2018; 18(1): 160.
[http://dx.doi.org/10.1186/s12905-018-0642-9] [PMID: 30285706]

[22]   Guyard A, Michelsen SI, Arnaud C, Fauconnier J. Family adaptation to cerebral palsy in adolescents: A European multicenter study. Res Dev Disabil 2017; 61: 138-50.
[http://dx.doi.org/10.1016/j.ridd.2016.11.010] [PMID: 28087202]

[23]   Adams JD. Risk factors for obesity.Cardiovascular and metabolic disease scientific discoveries and new therapies. London: Royal Society of Chemistry 2015; pp. 59-65.
[http://dx.doi.org/10.1039/9781782622390-00059]

[24]   Anderson SE, Keim SA. Parent-child interaction, self-regulation, and obesity prevention in early childhood. Curr Obes Rep 2016; 5(2): 192-200.
[http://dx.doi.org/10.1007/s13679-016-0208-9] [PMID: 27037572]

[25]   Tucker S, Lanningham-Foster LM. Nurse-led school-based child obesity prevention. J Sch Nurs 2015; 31(6): 450-66.jsn.sagepub.com
[http://dx.doi.org/10.1177/1059840515574002] [PMID: 25747899]

CHAPTER 4

Immunity and Balance

Abstract: The immune system depends on gut health and diet. Exercise, senescence and diseases also alter the homeostasis of the gut and other lymphoid tissues which affects the immune balance of the body. A healthy lifestyle is probably the most important therapy a patient can employ to maintain immune health.

Keywords: Alcohol, Autoimmunity, Diet, Exercise, Gut, Obesity, Senescence, Smoking.

1. INTRODUCTION

The body has many tissues that make up the immune system, skin, tonsils, adenoids, thymus, bronchus-associated lymphoid tissue, bone marrow, spleen, appendix and lymph nodes in various places. The immune system includes the Peyer's patches in the intestines, which are sites of maturation of many immune cells. Macrophages, T cells, B cells, M cells and dendritic cells in the Peyer's patches are critical to immune defenses against bacteria, viruses and fungi introduced into the gut.

Barriers such as the skin, GI tract, respiratory airways, nasopharynx, eyes and blood-brain barrier, are essential for keeping infectious organisms out of the body. The innate immune system prevents or limits infections by pathogens due to cellular immune recognition of danger-associated molecular patterns (DAMPs) produced on the plasma membranes of damaged cells [1]. Immune cells also recognize pathogen-associated molecular patterns (PAMPs) released by pathogenic bacteria and viruses. This means that recognition of DAMPs and PAMPs by immune cell pattern recognition receptors helps keep the body in balance and free of infections. Cells involved in the innate immune system include macrophages, mast cells, dendritic cells, natural killer cells and γδ T cells.

The adaptive immune system is activated once a pathogen enters the body [2]. B cells make antibodies that are part of the immunologic memory and are made for

James David Adams

specific non-self antigens. T cells secrete cytokines that help defeat invading pathogens. Stress is immunosuppressive, as has been discussed in the lifestyle chapter.

There is also a neuroimmune system that protects the brain from infections [3]. This involves T cells, B cells and the formation of antibodies and cytokines. The first line of defense of the brain is the blood-brain barrier that prevents most pathogens from entering the brain. In the brain, astrocytes, microglial cells, oligodendrocytes and mast cells protect neurons from infections and other damaging influences.

2. GUT HEALTH AND THE IMMUNE SYSTEM

Peyer's patches in the ileum, jejunum and duodenum are where the immune system can be directly influenced by diet. Pathogenic organisms in the gut are processed by macrophages, dendritic cells and M cells in the Peyer's patches [4]. This leads to T cell, B cell and memory cell activation near the Peyer's patches and immune cell amplification in mesenteric lymph nodes. Macrophages, dendritic cells and M cells have processes that directly contact the gut contents.

The Vagus nerve innervates the guts and is responsible for an anti-inflammatory effect through the activation of nicotinic receptors [NAChR, 5]. Vagal nerve stimulation decreases the production of TNF, IL-1β, IL-6 and IL-18. Gut myenteric neuron stimulation results from Vagal stimulation, blocks the activation of inflammatory Th17 cells, and activates anti-inflammatory Treg cells. There is a feedback mechanism to the brain involving peripheral IL-1 receptors on Vagal nerves.

The intestinal mucosa is persistently challenged by food and introduced allergens. A balance between defense and tolerance must be maintained. When this balance tips toward defense, pathology can occur, such as inflammatory bowel disease or Celiac Disease induced gluten intolerance. Vagal tone may be important in re-establishing tolerance and stopping inflammation. One of the most effective ways to increase vagal nerve outflow from the brain is by exercise. Smoking introduces nicotine into the guts and appears to decrease the severity of ulcerative colitis in patients [5]. Nicotine interacts with NAChR on Th2 cells and on nicotinic neurons [5] in this regard. However, several immune cells express NAChR, including macrophages, B cells, T cells and dendritic cells [5].

Decreased Vagal tone is a critical issue in heart patients and makes the heart less efficient. As Vagal tone decreases, inflammatory cytokines such as C-reactive protein are released by immune cells, gut cells and other cells. This leads to increased mortality in congestive heart failure [5].

3. DIET AND THE IMMUNE SYSTEM

Many flavonoids and other phenolic compounds have been reported to enhance immunity throughout the body. A number of these flavonoids are not well absorbed in the gut. It is critical to remember that dendritic cells, macrophages and M cells in the Peyer's patches come into contact with these compounds in the gut, even if they are not absorbed into the blood. These cells alter and enhance the gut immune response that affects the entire body. These compounds alter the immune system without being absorbed into the blood.

Humans have eaten vegetables and fruits for the entire span of our existence. Our bodies have responded and adapted to diet derived compounds. It is not surprising that plant derived flavonoids have become essential to our health and our immune health.

Chocolate contains several flavonols, including epicatechin (Fig. **1**) . Eating dark chocolate decreases blood pressure, increases flow mediated dilation and decreases insulin resistance [6]. Chocolate is also anti-inflammatory since it decreases adhesion molecule expression on leukocytes. Cocoa flavan-3-ols are cardioprotective since they decrease sE-selectin levels, a marker of leukocyte adhesion and endothelial function [6]. Epicatechin increases NO production, decreases blood glucose, insulin and insulin resistance [6]. Several genes involved in adipogenesis and inflammation are altered by epicatechin ingestion. It should be mentioned that a large portion of oral epicatechin is not absorbed in the intestines but is metabolized by gut microbes. These metabolites are absorbed into the blood and have pharmacological activities.

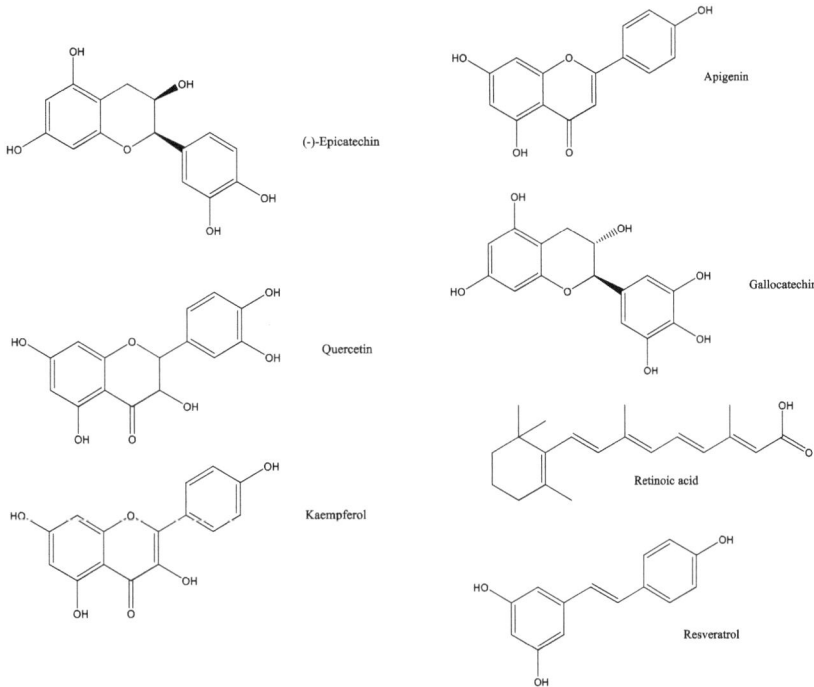

Fig. (1). Chemical structures of agents that alter gut immunity.

Flavonoids are helpful in upper respiratory tract infections since they enhance the gut immune system, which increases immunity throughout the body [7]. A systematic review and meta-analysis of 14 clinical trials found that flavonoid supplementation of 0.2 to 1.2 g per day resulted in decreased upper respiratory tract infections by 33% compared to placebo, with no adverse effects [7]. Athletes were similarly protected from infection in this study. Quercetin was one of the flavonoids used in this study (Fig. **1**) .

Quercetin has many beneficial effects in allergies and asthma, including inhibition of mast cell histamine release [8]. Quercetin ameliorates the symptoms of asthma and decreases asthma incidence. Apples, which contain quercetin, decrease childhood asthma when the mothers eat apples during pregnancy and decrease asthma incidence when eaten later in life [8]. In general, eating fruit increases lung health. This seems to be because flavonoids in fruit stimulate the gut immune system.

Cystic fibrosis is a serious disease of the lungs. Dietary flavonoids may be beneficial in patients suffering from cystic fibrosis [9]. Kaempferol, apigenin, gallocatechin (Fig. **1**) and flavonoid intake, in general, were found to be ameliorative in patients. These effects were mediated through the enhancement of the gut immune system.

People who eat more plant-derived foods and less meat tend to suffer less from cancer [10]. This is partly because red meat is known to increase cancer, as discussed in the lifestyle chapter. However, plant phenolics have anticancer activities. They work through NF-kB and AP-1 signaling cascades in cancer cells to kill cancer cells and decrease malignancy [10]. They also inhibit angiogenesis that is necessary for tumor growth and malignancy.

Resveratrol (Fig. **1**) has major effects on the immune system [11]. Fruit skins, such as grapes and blueberries are rich sources of resveratrol. The bioavailability of resveratrol is low [12]. Blood levels of resveratrol are not expected to reach pharmacologically active amounts. However, the actions of resveratrol in the gut, such as the Peyer's patches, are important. Macrophage anti-inflammatory activity is enhanced by resveratrol [11]. This may involve the inhibition of granulocyte macrophage colony-stimulating factor expression. As a result, cyclooxygenase-2 activity decreases in macrophages, which decreases prostaglandin production. T cell, CD4+ cell and Th17 cell activation is inhibited by resveratrol [11]. B cell activation decreases, as does antibody production. Low doses of resveratrol activate NK cells, whereas high doses inhibit NK cell activation [11].

Vitamin A deficiency is the primary cause of immune dysfunction in the world, especially T cell dysfunction [13]. Carotenes from plant sources and retinol from animal livers are major dietary sources of vitamin A or its precursors. Vitamin A has three forms, retinoic acid, retinal and retinol. Retinoic acid (Fig. **1**) is the major pharmacologically active form and exists as all-trans-retinoic acid and 9-cis-retinoic acid. They function by binding to retinoic acid receptors, retinoid X receptors and peroxisome proliferator-activated receptor β or δ. Retinoic acid stimulates gut homing of T cells, where they are further activated after initial activation in the lymph nodes [13]. Treg cell differentiation occurs after retinoic acid-binding and is important in maintaining the homeostasis of gut microbiota. T helper cell, Th1 and Th17, differentiation is inhibited by retinoic acid. Th2 cell functions are stimulated by retinoic acid [13].

Astaxanthin is a carotenoid found in fish and seafood [14]. Administration to young women resulted in a decrease in DNA damage and C reactive protein levels. T cell and B cell subpopulation changes occurred as well as alterations in the activities of other immune cells. Interferon-γ and IL-6 levels increased [14]. This demonstrates that even in healthy young women, carotenoid supplementation can alter immune cell activity.

Opuntia cacti come originally from the Americas. Various Opuntia species have been introduced around the world. Opuntia contains high levels of prebiotic fibers that enhance gut health and the gut microbiome [15]. It is critical not to destroy these dietary fibers by cooking. The best health benefits from cactus come from eating the pads or the fruit uncooked. Many clinical studies rely on cooked cactus that is of little benefit to health. The use of properly prepared Opuntia decreases blood glucose levels, blood insulin levels, and blood glucose-dependent insulinotropic peptides in diabetic patients [16]. Opuntia decreases inflammatory protein levels in the blood, including tumor necrosis factor α, IL-1β, IL-8, interferon γ and C reactive protein, and increases anti-inflammatory IL-10 [17].

4. EXERCISE AND IMMUNITY

As mentioned in the lifestyle chapter, exercise has profound effects on the body and generally increases health. Exercise strengthens the immune system, increases leukocytes in the circulation, and alters levels of several cytokines [18]. There are many effects of exercise on immune cells, Th1 cells decrease, NK cells increase, and lymphocytes increase. Exercise decreases severity and increases the survival of pneumonia and influenza [18]. The effects of exercise on the immune system are partly due to the effects of catecholamines released during exercise. In addition, immune cells synthesize dopamine that is used for the regulation of immune cells that have dopamine receptors [19].

Exercise benefits senescent people by stimulating their immune systems [18]. Elderly people suffer from a decline in the immune system called immunosenescence. This will be discussed later in this chapter. Exercise improves the levels of CD4+ and CD8+ cells in circulation in the elderly [18]. In addition, exercise increases anti-inflammatory cytokines such as IL-10 and decreases inflammatory cytokines such as IL-6 [18].

5. ALCOHOL

Gut health is compromised by alcohol and obesity, which affects immune health. Drinking too much alcohol leads to obesity since alcohol is an obesogen, as discussed in the lifestyle chapter. Chronic alcohol consumption is immunosuppressive and increases the risk of HIV, hepatitis C and *Mycobacterium tuberculosis* infection [20]. Alcohol alters the gut microbiome. Alcohol induces an inflammatory state in monocytes through a toll-like receptor mechanism and increases tumor necrosis factor α [20]. The inflammatory cytokine IL-1β increases due to alcohol, whereas the anti-inflammatory cytokine IL-10 decreases. Macrophages and neutrophils are activated by alcohol [20]. There is a shift in T helper cells to Th2 and Th17 responses. Dendritic cell functions are inhibited by alcohol.

Gut bacterial overgrowth can occur due to alcohol drinking [21]. Bacterial dysbiosis also occurs, which involves changes in good versus endotoxin-producing bacteria. Patients suffering from alcohol use disorder frequently have increased gut permeability [21]. This is due to damage to gut epithelial cells and the spaces between the cells. Alcohol metabolism in the gut, perhaps by the microsomal ethanol oxidizing system, produces oxygen radicals that damage epithelial cells. In addition, acetaldehyde produced during the metabolism of ethanol forms DNA adducts that damage DNA and can lead to cell death. Bacteria or endotoxins may leak out of the leaky gut leading to altered immune responses. Alcohol also damages Paneth cells, which secrete antimicrobial peptides [21]. Paneth cell damage allows bacterial overgrowth and endotoxin production. Leakage of endotoxins across the gut epithelium establishes an inflammatory reaction with T cell activation and inflammatory cytokine production.

Alcohol induced gut inflammation may enhance liver disease and gut cancer [21, 22]. Liver disease occurs in about 25% of heavy drinkers. There is also a gut brain axis where alteration of gut permeability and immune system leads to damage to the blood brain barrier and may be involved in the induction of Alzheimer's disease [23] and Parkinson's disease [24].

6. OBESITY

According to the WHO, one in ten adults is obese [25]. Obesity increases the risk of post-surgery infection, respiratory tract infection, periodontal infection, and nosocomial infection [25]. Intensive care unit patients who are obese are more likely to die than nonobese patients. During the 2009 H1N1 pandemic, obesity was associated with a worse outcome. Influenza is more likely to cause hospitalization in obese patients. A number of inflammatory adipokines are released from visceral fat cells during obesity. These adipokines have many effects on the immune system.

Leptin is an inflammatory adipokine that activates monocytes, neutrophils, Treg and NK cells [25]. The leptin receptor ObRb works through a JAK/STAT mechanism to affect immune cells. Monocyte and macrophage activation in visceral fat results in the secretion of IL-6, IL-1β, tumor necrosis factor α and monocyte chemoattractant protein-1 [26]. These inflammatory adipokines have effects on the heart, arteries, pancreas, joints and other tissues. This has been discussed in the lifestyle chapter.

Obesity increases the deposition of fat cells in lymphoid tissues like the bone marrow and thymus [26]. This results in less lymphoid progenitor cell proliferation and activation. CD4+ cells increase while CD8+ cells decrease. The gut microbiome is altered by obesity [27]. This gut dysbiosis is involved in obesity related non-alcoholic fatty liver disease and possibly other inflammatory conditions.

7. SENESCENCE AND THE IMMUNE SYSTEM

With age, immune responses decrease, leading to immune-aging and immune senescence. Changes in the immune system occur at the same time changes occur in muscles [28]. Sarcopenia occurs with aging and can account for a 2-4% loss of muscle strength per year. Type 2 fibers, also called fast-twitch fibers, are lost with aging. It is important to state that even in athletes that train daily, muscle loss occurs with aging. Exercise can slow down the loss of muscle as discussed earlier, but cannot stop or reverse the age-related loss of muscle. Insulin-like growth factor-1 is important in building muscle [28]. The actions of insulin-like growth factor-1 are inhibited by upregulation of protein kinase B (Akt) by mammalian target of rapamycin complex 2 (mTORC2). The activity of mTORC2 increases with aging [29].

As muscle tissue is lost, fat cells grow among the muscle fibers. This decreases the ability of the muscle to use insulin and can lead to insulin resistance [28]. Muscle is important in the clearance of blood insulin. Ectopic fat in muscle secretes inflammatory adipokines such as tumor necrosis factor α and IL-6. This inflammatory state is called inflammaging. Aging, IL-6 and tumor necrosis factor α cause 11β-hydroxysteroid dehydrogenase 1 activation [28], which increases blood cortisol levels. Cortisol accelerates muscle loss.

Neutrophils become activated in senescence but are less efficient due to Akt mTORC2 dysregulation [28]. These neutrophils establish an inflammatory state in tissues, such as muscle, that they infiltrate. Memory T cells and macrophages secrete more inflammatory cytokines in senescence. CD5+ B cells produce more autoantibodies with aging [30] while antibodies from other B cells in general decrease. Dendritic cells become less efficient, as do NK cells and macrophages. Age-associated thymus degeneration causes a decrease in T cell maturation, which results in fewer CD4 cells and CD8+ cells [30]. Blood cytokine levels are altered in senescence, with increases in inflammatory cytokines such as IL-6, C reactive protein, tumor necrosis factor α, and its soluble receptor 2 [31].

The gut microbiome also changes in senescence [32]. Many of the changes in the immune system may be the results of changes in the microbiome. There is a decrease in the number of Peyer's patches with aging that has major effects on T cell and B cell activation.

8. AUTOIMMUNE AND INFLAMMATORY DISEASES

The estrogen receptor is expressed in the cytoplasms of T cells, B cells, monocytes and dendrocytes [33]. The proliferation of B cells and T cells is inhibited by estrogen. However, B cells are activated by estrogen. T cell function such as IL-2 production is inhibited by estrogen. However, estrogen increases Th1 cell proliferation and interferon-γ production [33]. It also enhances Treg cell proliferation. An imbalance in estrogen effects has been implicated in autoimmune disorders such as systemic lupus erythematosus that affects women more than men [33]. Androgens and progestins are considered immunosuppressive in contrast to the immunostimulatory effects of estrogen in autoimmune disorders [33].

Gut diseases such as Crohn's disease and other inflammatory bowel diseases have effects on the immune system and could be caused by unbalanced immune responses [34]. In Crohn's disease T cell activation causes interferon-γ, tumor necrosis factor α and IL-23. Ulcerative colitis similarly involves T cell activation, but with IL-5 and IL-13 production. The T cells involved may be CD3+ T cells, although mast cells may also be activated [35]. T cell activation may be due to loss of regulation of T cells. This loss of regulation may involve toll-like receptors (TLR) expressed on intestinal epithelial cells [36]. TLR5 regulates intestinal microbiota and inflammation. TLR8 is upregulated in Crohn's disease and is involved in inflammatory mechanisms. TLR9 activation is protective in Crohn's disease patients [36].

Stress is an activator of inflammatory bowel diseases [37]. Stress increases corticotrophin-releasing factor, adrenocorticotropic hormone and cortisol. This alters the gut microbiota, alters gut permeability and activates mast cells. This may result in T cell activation or TLR alteration.

9. SMOKING

Smoking tobacco alters the functions of the immune system. Streptococcal pneumonia increases in smokers and second-hand smokers [38]. There is a lower respiratory tract microbiome that is involved in preventing lung infections. Smoking alters the lower respiratory tract microbiome, especially organisms in the Firmicutes and Proteobacteria groups, which may make smokers more prone to lung infections [39].

Lung resident mesenchymal stem cell immunomodulatory activity is decreased in smokers [40]. This results in altered cytokine production and decreased proliferation of CD8+ T cells. Cigarette smoke alters NFkB signaling, MAP kinase signaling and histone activity in immune cells [41].

This causes cellular dysfunction of macrophages, NK cells, alterations in TLRs on dendritic cells, dysfunction of Th1 cells, Th2 cells, Th17 cells, Treg cells, B cells and cytotoxic T cells. This immune dysfunction increases several diseases, including various cancers, rheumatoid arthritis, Crohn's disease and other autoimmune diseases [41]. Other diseases appear to increase in smokers, including Alzheimer's disease, Parkinson's disease, stroke and myocardial infarction [41].

CONCLUSIONS

The balance of the immune system is regulated in part by a neuroendocrine system, the hypothalamic oxytocin secreting system [42], which is part of the hypothalamo-neurohypophysial system. This system has neural connections throughout the brain and regulates other brain regions involved in maintaining the immune system. Oxytocin secreting neurons in this system can also secrete cytokines that affect the immune-modulating functions of other neurons. This, in turn, regulates the bone marrow, thymus and other lymphoid tissues. Not only does this involve the sympathetic nervous system, but also the limbic system [42], which is where emotions are processed. This implies that by self-regulating our emotions, we can regulate the balance of our immune systems to some extent.

REFERENCES

[1]   Gasteiger G, D'Osualdo A, Schubert DA, Weber A, Bruscia EM, Hartl D. Cellular innate immunity: An old game with new players. J Innate Immun 2017; 9(2): 111-25.
[http://dx.doi.org/10.1159/000453397] [PMID: 28006777]

[2]   Ito T, Connett JM, Kunkel SL, Matsukawa A. The linkage of innate and adaptive immune response during granulomatous development. Front Immunol 2013; 4: 10.
[http://dx.doi.org/10.3389/fimmu.2013.00010] [PMID: 23386849]

[3]   Dittel BN. CD4 T cells: Balancing the coming and going of autoimmune-mediated inflammation in the CNS. Brain Behav Immun 2008; 22(4): 421-30.
[http://dx.doi.org/10.1016/j.bbi.2007.11.010] [PMID: 18207698]

[4]   Wagner C, Bonnardel J, Da Silva C, Martens L, Gorvel JP, Lelouard H. Some news from the unknown soldier, the Peyer's patch macrophage. Cell Immunol 2018; 330: 159-67.
[http://dx.doi.org/10.1016/j.cellimm.2018.01.012] [PMID: 29395860]

[5]   Matteoli G, Boeckxstaens GE. The vagal innervation of the gut and immune homeostasis. Gut 2013; 62(8): 1214-22.
[http://dx.doi.org/10.1136/gutjnl-2012-302550] [PMID: 23023166]

[6]   Esser D, Geleijnse JM, Matualatupauw JC, *et al.* Pure flavonoid epicatechin and whole genome gene

expression profiles in circulating immune cells in adults with elevated blood pressure: A randomised double-blind, placebo-controlled, crossover trial. PLoS One 2018; 13(4)e0194229
[http://dx.doi.org/10.1371/journal.pone.0194229] [PMID: 29672527]

[7]   Somerville VS, Braakhuis AJ, Hopkins WG. Effect of flavonoids on upper respiratory tract infections and immune function: A systematic review and meta-analysis. Adv Nutr 2016; 7(3): 488-97.
[http://dx.doi.org/10.3945/an.115.010538] [PMID: 27184276]

[8]   Mlcek J, Jurikova T, Skrovankova S, Sochor J. Quercetin and its anti-allergic immune response. Molecules 2016; 21(5): 623.
[http://dx.doi.org/10.3390/molecules21050623] [PMID: 27187333]

[9]   Li L, Somerset S. Associations between flavonoid intakes and gut microbiota in a group of adults with cystic fibrosis. Nutrients 2018; 10(9): 1264.
[http://dx.doi.org/10.3390/nu10091264] [PMID: 30205496]

[10]   Wahle KW, Brown I, Rotondo D, Heys SD. Plant phenolics in the prevention and treatment of cancer. Adv Exp Med Biol 2010; 698: 36-51.
[http://dx.doi.org/10.1007/978-1-4419-7347-4_4] [PMID: 21520702]

[11]   Malaguarnera L. Influence of Resveratrol on the Immune Response. Nutrients 2019; 11(5): 946.
[http://dx.doi.org/10.3390/nu11050946] [PMID: 31035454]

[12]   Adams JD, Klaidman LK. Sirtuins, nicotinamide and aging: a critical review. Lett Drug Des Discov 2007; 4: 44-8.
[http://dx.doi.org/10.2174/157018007778992892]

[13]   Bono MR, Tejon G, Flores-Santibañez F, Fernandez D, Rosemblatt M, Sauma D. Retinoic acid as a modulator of T cell immunity. Nutrients 2016; 8(6): 349.
[http://dx.doi.org/10.3390/nu8060349] [PMID: 27304965]

[14]   Park JS, Chyun JH, Kim YK, Line LL, Chew BP. Astaxanthin decreased oxidative stress and inflammation and enhanced immune response in humans. Nutr Metab (Lond) 2010; 7: 18.http://www.nutritionandmetabolism.com/content/7/1/18
[http://dx.doi.org/10.1186/1743-7075-7-18] [PMID: 20205737]

[15]   Sánchez-Tapia M, Aguilar-López M, Pérez-Cruz C, *et al.* Nopal (Opuntia ficus indica) protects from metabolic endotoxemia by modifying gut microbiota in obese rats fed high fat/sucrose diet. Sci Rep 2017; 7(1): 4716.
[http://dx.doi.org/10.1038/s41598-017-05096-4] [PMID: 28680065]

[16]   López-Romero P, Pichardo-Ontiveros E, Avila-Nava A, *et al.* The effect of nopal (Opuntia ficus indica) on postprandial blood glucose, incretins, and antioxidant activity in Mexican patients with type 2 diabetes after consumption of two different composition breakfasts. J Acad Nutr Diet 2014; 114(11): 1811-8.
[http://dx.doi.org/10.1016/j.jand.2014.06.352] [PMID: 25132122]

[17]   Attanzio A, Tesoriere L, Vasto S, Pintaudi AM, Livrea MA, Allegra M. Short-term cactus pear [*Opuntia ficus-indica* (L.) Mill] fruit supplementation ameliorates the inflammatory profile and is associated with improved antioxidant status among healthy humans. Food Nutr Res 2018; 62.
[http://dx.doi.org/10.29219/fnr.v62.1262] [PMID: 30150921]

[18]   Pelinski da Silveira M, da Silva Fagundes K, Ribeiro Bizuti M, Starck E, Calciolari Rossi R. Physical exercise as a tool to help the immune system against COVID 19: an integrative review of the current literature. Clin Exp Med 2021; 21: 15-28.
[http://dx.doi.org/10.1007/s10238-020-00650-3]

[19]   Kawano M, Takagi R, Saika K, Matsui M, Matsushita S. Dopamine regulates cytokine secretion during innate and adaptive immune responses. Int Immunol 2018; 30(12): 591-606.
[http://dx.doi.org/10.1093/intimm/dxy057] [PMID: 30165447]

[20]   Szabo G, Saha B. Alcohol's effect on host defense. Alcohol Res 2015; 37(2): 159-70.

[PMID: 26695755]

[21]   Bishehsari F, Magno E, Swanson G, *et al.* Alcohol and gut-derived inflammation. Alcohol Res 2017; 38(2): 163-71.
[PMID: 28988571]

[22]   Dubinkina VB, Tyakht AV, Odintsova VY, *et al.* Links of gut microbiota composition with alcohol dependence syndrome and alcoholic liver disease. Microbiome 2017; 5(1): 141-55.
[http://dx.doi.org/10.1186/s40168-017-0359-2] [PMID: 29041989]

[23]   Adams J. Can peripheral inflammation cause Alzheimer's disease? Biomed Res J 2019; 1: 1-3.

[24]   Lien E, Adams J, Lien L, Law M. Parkinson's disease: in search of the means of prevention and treatment. Ann Clin Pharmacol Ther 2019; 2: 1-5.

[25]   Milner JJ, Beck MA. The impact of obesity on the immune response to infection. Proc Nutr Soc 2012; 71(2): 298-306.
[http://dx.doi.org/10.1017/S0029665112000158] [PMID: 22414338]

[26]   Andersen CJ, Murphy KE, Fernandez ML. Impact of obesity and metabolic syndrome on immunity. Adv Nutr 2016; 7(1): 66-75.
[http://dx.doi.org/10.3945/an.115.010207] [PMID: 26773015]

[27]   Marchesi JR, Adams DH, Fava F, *et al.* The gut microbiota and host health: a new clinical frontier. Gut 2016; 65(2): 330-9.
[http://dx.doi.org/10.1136/gutjnl-2015-309990] [PMID: 26338727]

[28]   Wilson D, Jackson T, Sapey E, Lord JM. Frailty and sarcopenia: The potential role of an aged immune system. Ageing Res Rev 2017; 36: 1-10.
[http://dx.doi.org/10.1016/j.arr.2017.01.006] [PMID: 28223244]

[29]   Chellappa K, Brinkman JA, Mukherjee S, *et al.* Hypothalamic mTORC2 is essential for metabolic health and longevity. Aging Cell 2019; 18(5)e13014
[http://dx.doi.org/10.1111/acel.13014] [PMID: 31373126]

[30]   Fuentes E, Fuentes M, Alarcón M, Palomo I. Immune system dysfunction in the elderly. An Acad Bras Cienc 2017; 89(1): 285-99.
[http://dx.doi.org/10.1590/0001-3765201720160487] [PMID: 28423084]

[31]   Marcos-Pérez D, Sánchez-Flores M, Maseda A, *et al.* Frailty in older adults Is associated with plasma concentrations of inflammatory mediators but not with lymphocyte subpopulations. Front Immunol 2018; 9: 1056.
[http://dx.doi.org/10.3389/fimmu.2018.01056] [PMID: 29868017]

[32]   García-Peña C, Álvarez-Cisneros T, Quiroz-Baez R, Friedland RP. Microbiota and aging. A review and commentary. Arch Med Res 2017; 48(8): 681-9.
[http://dx.doi.org/10.1016/j.arcmed.2017.11.005] [PMID: 29229199]

[33]   Moulton VR. Sex hormones in acquired immunity and autoimmune disease. Front Immunol 2018; 9: 2279.
[http://dx.doi.org/10.3389/fimmu.2018.02279] [PMID: 30337927]

[34]   Huibregtse IL, van Lent AU, van Deventer SJ. Immunopathogenesis of IBD: insufficient suppressor function in the gut? Gut 2007; 56(4): 584-92.
[http://dx.doi.org/10.1136/gut.2006.103523] [PMID: 17047100]

[35]   Bashashati M, Moossavi S, Cremon C, *et al.* Colonic immune cells in irritable bowel syndrome: A systematic review and meta-analysis. Neurogastroenterol Motil 2018; 30(1)e13192
[http://dx.doi.org/10.1111/nmo.13192] [PMID: 28851005]

[36]   Lu Y, Li X, Liu S, Zhang Y, Zhang D. Toll-like receptors and inflammatory bowel disease. Front Immunol 2018; 9: 72.
[http://dx.doi.org/10.3389/fimmu.2018.00072] [PMID: 29441063]

[37]   Qin HY, Cheng CW, Tang XD, Bian ZX. Impact of psychological stress on irritable bowel syndrome. World J Gastroenterol 2014; 20(39): 14126-31.
[http://dx.doi.org/10.3748/wjg.v20.i39.14126] [PMID: 25339801]

[38]   Almirall J, Blanquer J, Bello S. Community-acquired pneumonia among smokers. Arch Bronconeumol 2014; 50(6): 250-4.
[http://dx.doi.org/10.1016/j.arbres.2013.11.016] [PMID: 24387877]

[39]   Li KJ, Chen ZL, Huang Y, *et al.* Dysbiosis of lower respiratory tract microbiome are associated with inflammation and microbial function variety. Respir Res 2019; 20(1): 272.
[http://dx.doi.org/10.1186/s12931-019-1246-0] [PMID: 31796027]

[40]   Cruz T, López-Giraldo A, Noell G, *et al.* Smoking impairs the immunomodulatory capacity of lung-resident mesenchymal stem cells in chronic obstructive pulmonary disease. Am J Respir Cell Mol Biol 2019; 61(5): 575-83.
[http://dx.doi.org/10.1165/rcmb.2018-0351OC] [PMID: 30978114]

[41]   Qiu F, Liang CL, Liu H, *et al.* Impacts of cigarette smoking on immune responsiveness: Up and down or upside down? Oncotarget 2017; 8(1): 268-84.
[http://dx.doi.org/10.18632/oncotarget.13613] [PMID: 27902485]

[42]   Li T, Wang P, Wang SC, Wang YF. Approaches mediating oxytocin regulation of the immune system. Front Immunol 2017; 7: 693.
[http://dx.doi.org/10.3389/fimmu.2016.00693] [PMID: 28119696]

CHAPTER 5

The Endocannabinoid System and Balance

Abstract: The endocannabinoid system is a complex, redundant system that maintains the balance of normal health. It is a part of the eicosanoid system and interacts extensively with various eicosanoids and their receptors. Imbalance in the endocannabinoid/eicosanoid system leads to diseases that can be chronic and life-threatening, such as pain, diabetes, epilepsy and post-traumatic stress disorder. Plant-based medicines can be used to reestablish the necessary balance and effectively treat these disorders. However, it is always best to live in balance and allow the body to heal itself.

Keywords: Anxiety, Arthritis, Autism, Cancer, Cannabinoids, Chronic Ain, Chronic Fatigue Syndrome, Eicosanoids, Epilepsy, HIV/ADIS, Irritable Bowel Syndrome, Migraines, Multiple Sclerosis, Obesity, Pain, Post-traumatic Stress Disorder, Psoriasis, Traumatic Brain Injury, Type 2 Diabetes.

1. INTRODUCTION

The endocannabinoid system, endocannabinoidome, consists of endocannabinoids, the synthetic enzymes that make them, the enzymes that degrade them, and the receptors they interact with [1]. The endocannabinoids (Fig. **1**) are N-arachidonoyl ethanolamine (anandamide) and 2-arachidonoylglycerol (2AG). Endocannabinoids are involved in homeostasis at the cellular and organ levels. Disruption of this balance is critical to several diseases. The endocannabinoidome is involved in cognition, fertility, pregnancy, fetal development, infant development, immune functions, appetite, pain, memory, mood and other functions.

Since the endocannabinoid system is critical to health, the body has several redundant pathways for the synthesis and degradation of endocannabinoids [1]. Receptor promiscuity is another hallmark of the system; in other words, an agonist for one specialized receptor, such as a prostaglandin receptor, may interact with another specialized receptor, such as an endocannabinoid receptor. This makes the system very complex and difficult to manipulate with agonists or antagonists.

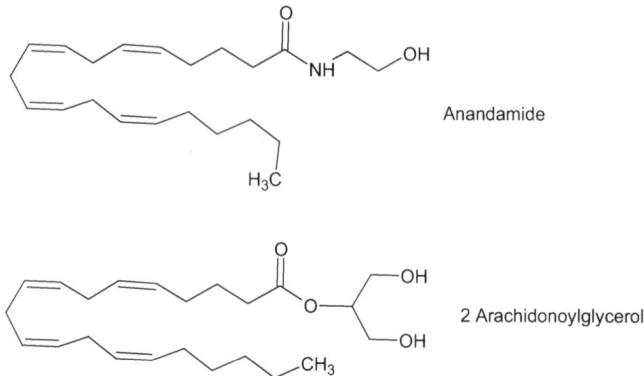

Fig. (1). Endocannabinoids.

The receptors that endocannabinoids interact with include cannabinoid receptor 1 (CB1), cannabinoid receptor 2 (CB2) and several other receptors. CB1 and CB2 are G-protein coupled receptors. Most CB1 receptors in the brain are presynaptic, but some postsynaptic and astrocytic CB1 receptors have been reported [2]. CB1 presynaptic receptors inhibit the release of glutamate and γ-aminobutyric acid (GABA). Endocannabinoids also interact with transient receptor potential cation channels. CB1 is most abundant in the brain, but is also found in many other tissues [1]. CB1 receptor activation is involved in dysbiosis, an imbalance of gut bacteria that can be accompanied by increased intestinal permeability. CB2 is primarily found on immune cells but is found on microglia and other places as well. CB2 receptors are involved in the regulation of leakage across the blood-brain barrier [1].

The enzyme that makes anandamide is N-acylphosphatidylethanolamine specific phospholipase D like hydrolase (NAPEPLD). This enzyme makes other N-acylethanolamines as well [1]. Some of these are putative endocannabinoids. Anandamide is made upon demand in the postsynaptic terminal, is released into the synapse, where it acts on presynaptic CB1 receptors and is degraded. There is no vesicular storage of anandamide. Anandamide is an agonist for CB1, CB2, peroxisome proliferator-activated receptor γ, and an antagonist for Cav3.2 calcium channel, transient receptor potential cation channel vanilloid 1 (TRPV1), and TRP melastatin 8 (TRPM8). It is both an agonist and an antagonist for TRPV1 since long-term activation leads to inhibition.

Brain TRPV1 binding by endocannabinoids stimulates hunger, fear, anxiety, and memory [1]. The activation of brain peroxisome proliferator-activated receptor (PPAR) α and γ by endocannabinoids is neuroprotective and anti-inflammatory.

The enzyme that degrades anandamide is fatty acid amide hydrolase (FAAH) which is a membrane-bound enzyme. This enzyme also degrades other N-acylethanolamines and fatty acid amides [1]. The enzyme works very rapidly to degrade anandamide and stop its actions.

The synthesis of monoacylglycerols, including 2AG, is catalyzed by diacylglyercol lipase α and β [1]. This occurs on-demand in the postsynaptic terminal. There is no vesicular storage of 2AG. The release of 2AG into the synapse allows it to interact with presynaptic CB1 receptors. 2AG is a more effective agonist for CB1 than anandamide. 2AG is degraded rapidly by monoacylglycerol lipase, a membrane-associated enzyme. Other receptors that 2AG is an agonist for include TRPV1 and $GABA_A$. 2AG and anandamide are also broken down by cyclooxygenase-2, which means that inhibition of cyclooxygenase-2, such as by nonsteroidal anti-inflammatory drugs increases endocannabinoids and decreases prostaglandins [2].

Several endogenous compounds interact with the endocannabinoid system. N-Acyl-dopamines, fatty acid primary amides, N-acyl-serotonins, N-acyl-taurines and N-acyl-amino acids all have their own receptors but can also interact with endocannabinoid receptors. This contributes to the complexity and redundancy of the endocannabinoid system.

2. OBESITY

Endocannabinoids are made by visceral fat and secreted into the blood [3]. They act on visceral fat cells as paracrine mediators to decrease adiponectin production and increase the production of inflammatory adipokines, including visfatin and tumor necrosis factor α. These adipokines are involved in causing several diseases, as discussed in the lifestyle chapter. This demonstrates the importance of living in balance. Too much endocannabinoid synthesis in obesity produces a proinflammatory condition. The right amount of endocannabinoids is required for normal health.

3. PROSTAGLANDINS AND OTHER EICOSANOIDS

Arachidonic acid is the starting material for endocannabinoids, isoprostanes, prostaglandins, leukotrienes, thromboxanes, lipoxins and other compounds (Fig. **2 - 5**). All of these eicosanoids exist in a balance. When the body needs prostaglandins, the synthesis of other eicosanoids may decrease. When the demand for endocannabinoids increases in an organ, the synthesis of other eicosanoids may decrease temporarily. Some eicosanoids are kept separate from others due to the sites of synthesis. For instance, thromboxanes are made in platelets but are secreted into the plasma. Prostaglandins are made in platelets and other cells. These eicosanoids have their own receptors but sometimes can activate receptors for other eicosanoids. For instance, prostaglandins have their own prostaglandin receptors but can also transactivate through phosphorylation, endocannabinoid TRP channels [4].

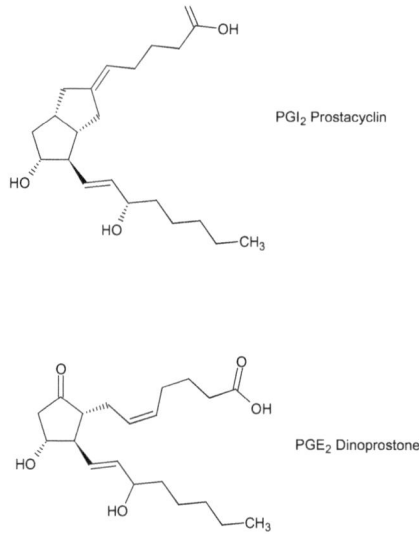

PGI$_2$ Prostacyclin

PGE$_2$ Dinoprostone

Fig. (2). Prostaglandins.

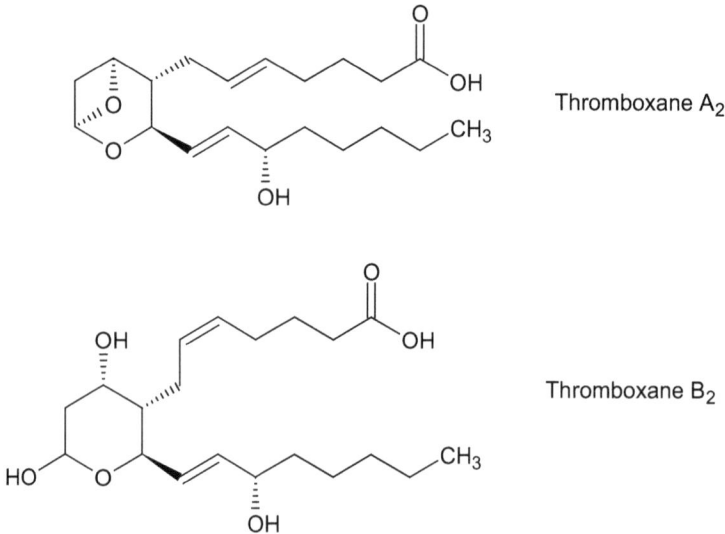

Thromboxane A$_2$

Thromboxane B$_2$

Fig. (3). Thromboxanes.

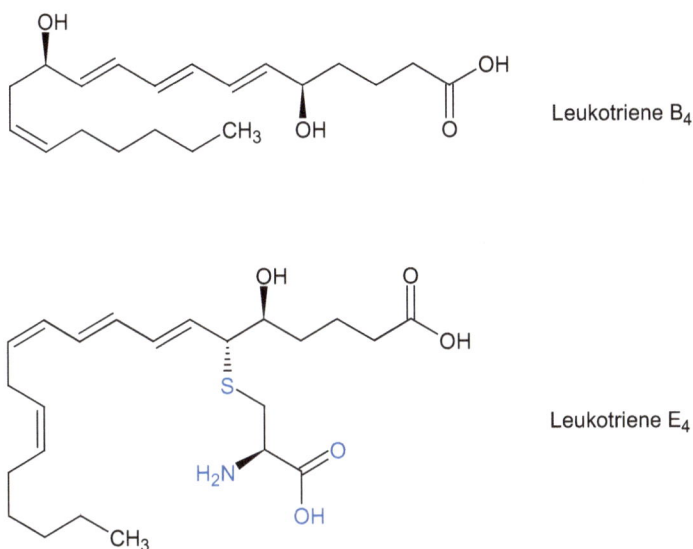

Leukotriene B4

Leukotriene E4

Fig. (4). Leukotrienes.

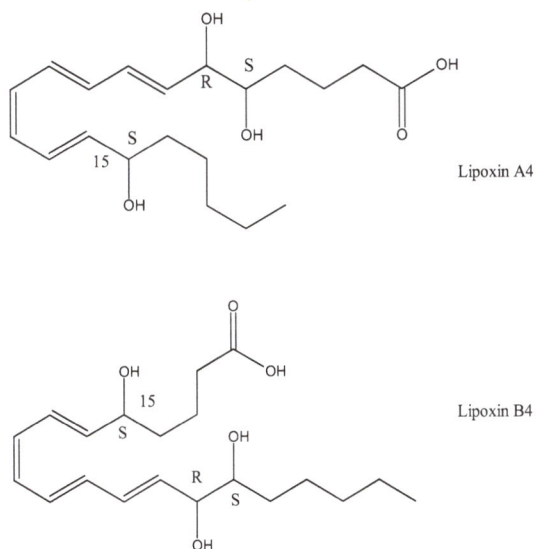

Lipoxin A4

Lipoxin B4

Fig. (5). Lipoxins.

Several drugs, nonsteroidal anti-inflammatory drugs are used to decrease prostaglandin production by inhibition of cyclooxygenase 1 and 2. Inhibition of prostaglandin E2 production should decrease pain. However, inhibition of prostacyclin production by these drugs increases clotting. Decreased prostacyclin decreases sirtuin-1 and PPARδ expression, and increases the expression of tissue factor, the major thrombosis initiating factor [5]. This increases clotting events, including heart attacks and strokes. That is why the FDA issued a warning about increased clotting with these drugs in July of 2015. These drugs are estimated by the FDA to increase clotting by 10 to 50%, which may be as many as 55,000 deaths yearly from heart attacks and strokes in the US.

Specific inhibition of cyclooxygenase 2 by celecoxib and acetaminophen, does not decrease thromboxane production by cyclooxygenase 1 [6]. This can lead to thrombosis. Of course, decreased prostacyclin production by these drugs also enhances thrombosis, as above.

Prostaglandins have an inflammatory activity, which may be important in asthma and cancer. Prostaglandin E2 is involved in tumor growth by acting through its receptor, prostaglandin E receptor 4, EP4 [7]. Prostaglandin E2 inhibits the antitumor actions of natural killer cells, decreases the antitumor actions of CD8+ T cells and inhibits the supply of dendritic cell precursors to the tumor, which is involved in antigen presentation to immune cells. Inhibition of EP4 may be an approach to improve cell killing in cancer.

Prostaglandin D2 receptor 2, DP2, is involved in lung inflammation in asthma [8]. DP2 activity increases eosinophil activation, the release of several inflammatory cytokines and increases airway muscle mass. Antagonism of DP2 may be useful in the treatment of asthma.

4. PAIN AND CHRONIC PAIN

Pain is created in the skin as a warning of potential harm that might occur unless the harmful stimulus is avoided. The skin is the pain-sensing organ and helps defend the body against harm. Sensory neurons in the skin use TRP channels to sense pain [4]. Endocannabinoids are produced rapidly to cause pain. A few minutes after the painful stimulus is removed, the TRP channels become deactivated by endocannabinoids and pain subsides. This makes TRP channels uniquely useful for pain sensation, the agonists that activate them also deactivate them. TRP channel activation can also cause capillary leakage leading to edema in the skin.

Pain and chronic pain involve multiple components of the eicosanoid system: endocannabinoids, prostaglandins, leukotrienes, lipoxins and resolvins [4]. Endocannabinoids cause initial pain. There is a complex interaction between these systems that is increased by the actions of chemokines [9, 10]. Chemokines are secreted by sensory neurons and attract macrophages into the skin that make prostaglandins due to the actions of cyclo-oxygenase-2. Macrophages release chemokines that activate TRP channels, enhancing pain. Chemokines also attract neutrophils into the skin that make leukotrienes. In a slow and long-term process, TRP channels are activated by leukotrienes with no deactivation of TRP channels, perhaps involving phosphorylation of TRP channels. Bradykinins are released into the skin following damage and enhance pain by increasing chemokine production, activating TRP channels. Chemokines turn the skin into a pain-producing organ. This pain chemokine cycle is the basis of chronic pain. Inhibiting chemokine production in the skin cures chronic pain [11].

Activation of TRP channels causes sensory neurons to release neurokinins, which are inflammatory proteins [10]. These proteins enhance inflammation at sites that are at risks, such as arthritic joints or damaged ligaments. Pain leads to inflammation.

The treatment of pain and chronic pain is most efficacious with topical products that contain monoterpenoids [9 - 11]. Topical tetrahydrocannabinol (THC) or cannabidiol (CBD) may also help [12]. THC is an agonist for CB1 receptors and an agonist/deactivator of TRP channels. Skin CB1 receptor activation decreases pain [4]. CBD is a CB1 antagonist and an agonist/deactivator of TRP channels. Monoterpenoids have the advantage that they penetrate into the skin, inhibit TRP channels relieving pain, and evaporate from the skin. They do not have to be absorbed into the blood to be effective. This greatly limits any toxicity from monoterpenoids.

5. CANNABINOIDS AND ENDOCANNABINOIDS

Plant-derived cannabinoids interact with the endocannabinoid system. THC tolerance in chronic marijuana smokers decreases CB1 expression [12]. Marijuana is *Cannabis sativa*. The name marijuana comes from the Chinese name for the plant Ma (hemp), Ren (seed), Hua (flower). CBD inhibits FAAH and blocks the reuptake of anandamide [12]. The chronic effect of smoking marijuana high in THC is to decrease the effects of the endocannabinoid system. The use of CBD products may enhance the effects of anandamide.

6. ANXIETY AND ENDOCANNABINOIDS

It is estimated that as many as 12% of people suffer from anxiety such as phobias, social anxiety, or panic disorders. Anxiety involves fear learning which is an exaggerated emotional response to perceived danger. Endocannabinoids activate brain CB1, which inhibits GABA release, possibly stopping anxiety. GABA receptor inhibition by benzodiazepines relieves anxiety. Endocannabinoids activate then deactivate brain TRPV1 channels [13]. This may relieve anxiety.

However, smoking marijuana rich in THC increases anxiety [14]. This is because chronic marijuana use downregulates CB1 receptors and may increase GABA release. CBD may decrease anxiety [15], perhaps since CBD is a partial agonist for the serotonin 1A receptor. Some patients have found that using topical CBD preparations on the neck or face provides effective anxiety relief. This may be because of serotonin 1A receptor activation in the skin.

7. AUTISM

Autism spectrum disorders (ASD) have increased 3-fold in the last 3 decades. Males are affected 4 times more than females. This condition develops in childhood and appears to be caused by risk factors present in the parents. Parental risk factors include age greater than 30, family history of the condition, maternal gestational diabetes, maternal use of acetaminophen, valproic acid, or selective serotonin reuptake inhibitors during pregnancy [16, 17].

Valproic acid alters brain GABA levels and may alter brain connections through a GABAergic mechanism. It also increases FAAH transcription and endocannabinoid levels [18]. Selective serotonin reuptake inhibitors alter brain serotonin levels and increase the effects of endocannabinoids [19, 20].

Acetaminophen is a selective cyclo-oxygenase 2 inhibitor that increases endocannabinoid synthesis [21, 22]. It is also metabolized to N-arachidonoylaminophenol that activates CB1 receptors and is an activator/deactivator for TRPV1; in other words, it acts like an endocannabinoid. It is possible that increased endocannabinoid activity in the fetal brain due to maternal acetaminophen use is a major cause of ASD. It is also possible that the use of acetaminophen in infancy increases the risk of developing ASD.

Connectivity between brain regions is abnormal in ASD, increased in some areas, decreased in others. These connections depend on cell adhesion molecules. The proteins that anchor cell adhesion molecules, catenins, have been reported to be mutated in ASD [23]. Catenins interact with endocannabinoids in memory extinction [24] which may be important in ASD. Mutated catenins may not be able to interact correctly with endocannabinoids.

The gut is involved in ASD, with 70% of patients experiencing chronic gut disorders [25]. This may alter the immune system, which depends on the gut, and lead to an inflammatory state in the brain and other sites during development.

Microglial cells, which have immune functions in the brain, have been reported to be overly active in ASD [23].

Several clinical reports have found that CBD improves symptoms and quality of life in ASD [26, 27]. A case study found that cannabidiolic acid is even better than CBD for ASD [28]. There are a few possible mechanisms of action of CBD in ASD. CBD increases brain endocannabinoids [29], which are low in ASD [30], despite possibly being elevated in the fetal or infant's brain. CBD also decreases gut leakage, which may help decrease inflammation in ASD [31].

8. CANCER

Some cancers are associated with high tumor endocannabinoids, CB1 and CB2, such as skin, prostate, colon, hepatocellular, endometrial sarcoma, glioblastoma multiforme, meningioma, pituitary adenoma and Hodgkin's lymphoma [32]. However, it is not clear that any cancers are caused by endocannabinoids.

Cancer is associated with pain. Cancer chemotherapy is associated with nausea. Both pain and nausea are sometimes treated with marijuana, dronabinol, nabilone and nabiximols. All of these treatments have been tested in clinical trials and found to be effective [33]. Unwanted side effects include dizziness, dysphoria, hallucinations, depression, paranoia and hypotension. These compounds can also stimulate appetite in cancer patients but are not as good as megestrol.

9. CHRONIC FATIGUE SYNDROME

Myalgic encephalomyelitis or chronic fatigue syndrome is associated with chronic fatigue, chronic pain, irritable bowel syndrome and other symptoms. Blood levels of natural killer cells, complement and IL-10 are high in the disease [34]. Brain neuroinflammation is prominent [35]. Chronic fatigue syndrome differs from fibromyalgia due to prominent fatigue and bowel issues.

Rintatolimod, the Toll-like receptor 3 agonist, is ineffective in chronic fatigue syndrome [36], as is rituximab [37]. Rituximab binds to B-lymphocyte antigen CD-20 and decreases the ability of natural killer cells to kill B cells.

It has been proposed that in chronic fatigue syndrome, endocannabinoids interact with TRPV1 receptors to generate oxygen radicals and make the blood brain barrier leaky [38]. This attracts natural killer cells into the brain and leads to neuroinflammation. It is also possible that initial damage to muscles stimulates chemokine production that attracts macrophages, activates natural killer cells and increases IL-10 release from muscles. This may lead to chronic pain in the muscles.

CBD decreases the leakiness of the blood brain barrier and inhibits TRPV1 [39]. CBD also decreases gut leakiness and may be helpful in chronic gut disorders associated with chronic fatigue syndrome [31]. CBD should be tested in clinical trials against chronic fatigue syndrome.

10. TYPE 2 DIABETES

Obesity is the cause of type 2 diabetes in 85% of patients, as discussed in the lifestyle chapter. Retinopathy occurs in 50% of these patients [40]. Nephropathy is observed in 30% of these patients. Type 2 diabetes accounts for 60% of all limb amputations. Patients would rather lose a leg than change their lifestyles. The way to cure type 2 diabetes is through living in balance, as described in the lifestyle chapter.

CB1 and CB2 are found in the pancreas. CB1 stimulation by endocannabinoids causes insulin and glucagon secretion [41]. CB2 stimulation decreases insulin secretion. CB1 excessive activation in the pancreas and other sites has been linked to reactive oxygen species generation leading to endothelial dysfunction [42]. Endothelial damage causes retinopathy, atherosclerosis, nephropathy and gangrene. CB2 over-stimulation in the pancreas and other sites causes leukocyte adhesion and activation in arterioles and arteries, enhancing endothelial dysfunction.

Marijuana smoking is an effective way to prevent type 2 diabetes in some people. Marijuana smokers have smaller waist circumferences, less obesity, less metabolic syndrome, lower fasting insulin, less insulin resistance and lower blood glucose than controls [43, 44]. There is no evidence that marijuana smoking causes type 2 diabetes [45]. Marijuana smokers exhibit CB1 downregulation leading to lower inflammatory adipokine secretion into the blood [46].

11. EPILEPSY

Epilepsy is a chronic disease that usually begins in childhood. The endocannabinoid system is altered in epilepsy. 2AG synthesis can be low in epilepsy due to the low activity of diacylglycerol lipase α [47]. Astrocytic cyclooxygenase-2 is elevated in epilepsy and increases the catabolism of 2AG and anandamide. Low endocannabinoid levels in some synapses due to astrocytic catabolism, may be important in epilepsy. CB1 receptors are increased in cholecystokininergic neurons that synapse with inhibitory GABAergic neurons, while they are decreased in excitatory neurons that synapse with glutamatergic neurons in epilepsy. This creates too little inhibitory activity and too much excitatory activity leading to seizures.

It is possible that inhibition of CB1 receptors, such as with CBD, may reestablish the balance of excitatory and inhibitory neuronal activity in the brain and decrease seizures. CBD interacts with other receptors that may be important in epilepsy, such as TRPV1, orphan G protein-coupled receptor 55, and equilibrative nucleoside transporter 1. CBD has been approved for use in some intractable seizures such as Lennox-Gastaut syndrome and Dravet syndrome. There is insufficient evidence for the use of CBD in other forms of epilepsy.

Diet can decrease seizures. A high fat, low carbohydrate diet can prevent seizures [48]. The diet should be vegetarian since eating meat in high fat, low carbohydrate diet for more than 6 months increases all-cause mortality [48, 49].

12. HIV/AIDS

The human immunodeficiency virus (HIV) suppresses CD4+ T cells which allows HIV to proliferate. Weight loss, anorexia, an acquired immunodeficiency syndrome (AIDS) and AIDS dementia can be problematic in these patients. HIV-1 envelope glycoprotein GP120 is toxic to cortical neurons [50]. Transactivator of transcription, a protein secreted by HIV, is toxic to cortical neurons [51]. These toxic proteins may lead to AIDS dementia. Endocannabinoid activation of CB1 appears to inhibit both of these neurotoxicities.

AIDS patients smoke marijuana to treat their symptoms. There is insufficient evidence that marijuana helps with anorexia, weight gain, or mortality in AIDS [52]. There are no reports of the effects of marijuana on AIDS dementia. AIDS patients should be aware that smoking marijuana may increase opportunistic infections and should use marijuana in moderation.

13. IRRITABLE BOWEL SYNDROME

Irritable bowel syndrome is a chronic inflammation of the gut involving increased enterochromaffin cells, intraepithelial lymphocytes, and mast cells [5, 53]. The condition is marked by attacks and remissions. Several drugs, including hyoscyamine, are used to treat, but not cure, the syndrome.

The gut contains over 100 million neurons, many of which are regulated by endocannabinoids [5, 53]. Endocannabinoids are CB1 agonists and decrease propulsion, secretions and increase leakiness. They also regulate gut mast cells through CB1 receptor activation. Anandamide and 2AG are TRPV1 agonists and can increase inflammation before TRPV1 becomes deactivated. TRPV1 is increased 3.5 fold in the gut in irritable bowel syndrome [54]. This indicates that TRPV1 is important in disease causation and treatment. The enzyme that synthesizes 2AG, diacylglycerol lipase α, is increased in the gut epithelium in irritable bowel syndrome. The enzyme that catabolizes 2AG, monoacylglycerol lipase, is increased as well. The enzyme that synthesizes anandamide, NAPEPLD, is decreased in the gut epithelium in the syndrome and results in decreased anandamide.

Peppermint oil has been shown in several studies and a meta-analysis to be an effective treatment of irritable bowel syndrome [53 - 55]. Peppermint oil contains cineole, menthol, and other monoterpenoids that are TRPV1 activators/deactivators. This may be why after dinner, mints are popular.

Fecal transplants are the only reported cures for irritable bowel syndrome. Probiotics have been found to be useful. Diet modification is also useful [53, 55], especially temporary cessation of fiber, oligo-, di- monosaccharides and polyols, which come from barley, wheat, rye, vegetables, and fruit. Long-term cessation of these nutrients is detrimental.

There is no evidence that THC or marijuana is helpful in the treatment of irritable bowel syndrome [53, 55]. However, cannabidiol is helpful since it inhibits TRPV1 and decreases gut leakiness [56].

14. MIGRAINES

Migraine headaches are produced by vasodilation of arterioles in the skin of the head through TRP melastatin 8 (TRPM8) receptor activation in the skin [57, 58]. Old theories that migraines are generated in the brain and brainstem are not viable since the brain does not directly feel pain. Both THC and CBD are activator/deactivators for TRPM8 [12]. Many migraine patients smoke marijuana in an attempt to prevent their migraines.

Smoking marijuana can decrease the frequency of migraines from 10.4 to 4.6 per month, with the majority of patients reporting favorable results [59]. It is possible that using topical THC, CBD or monoterpenoids to inhibit TRPM8 will be a faster and more effective way to treat migraines. Cannabinoids that inhibit peripheral TRPA1 (TRP ankyrin1) are useful in a rodent model of migraines, which suggests that migraines may be caused by TRPA1 activation as well as TRPM8 activation [60].

15. MULTIPLE SCLEROSIS

Multiple sclerosis is caused by progressive demyelination of nerves in the brain and brain stem leading to permanent neurological problems. Demyelination is due to the body's own immune cells attacking myelin [61]. This involves T cells, B cells and macrophages. The blood brain barrier becomes more permeable in the disease. CB2 receptor stimulation by endocannabinoids or THC has been proposed to inhibit immune cell activity in multiple sclerosis and may be beneficial. However, dronabinol is not effective at alleviating disease symptoms or progression [61].

Oral marijuana extracts and oral THC have been reported to relieve muscle stiffness, pain, spasms and improve sleep in multiple sclerosis [62]. Oral nabiximols have also been found to decrease spasticity, spasms and increase sleep quality [63]. Nabiximols contain equal amounts of THC and CBD, as well as peppermint oil. Nabiximols are standard therapy for multiple sclerosis in many countries. Diroximel fumarate is also available and is an immunomodulatory agent that decreases relapses and lesions.

16. OSTEOARTHRITIS, RHEUMATOID ARTHRITIS

Osteoarthritis is caused by endocannabinoids and adipokines released from visceral fat in obesity, as discussed in the lifestyle chapter. Rheumatoid arthritis is caused by adipokine secretion in the synovium by fibroblast-like synoviocytes, B cells and macrophages [64 - 66]. IL-6 and tumor necrosis factor α produced by fibroblast-like synoviocytes stimulate adipokine secretion. This process leads to osteoclast formation from macrophages. Endocannabinoids stimulate CB2 on fibroblast-like synoviocytes and inhibit adipokine production. CB1 antagonists and CB2 agonists inhibit osteoclast formation.

Marijuana could be useful in osteoarthritis and rheumatoid arthritis in part from CB2 receptor stimulation. However, there is no evidence that marijuana-based treatments are effective [67]. There are at least 5 clinical trials of marijuana-based products ongoing, however. As stated above, smoking marijuana down regulates CB1 receptors, endocannabinoid synthesis and adipokine synthesis [46]. This should be beneficial in osteoarthritis and rheumatoid arthritis. Topical THC, CBD and monoterpenoids can help with pain and inflammation in these conditions [4]. The way to cure osteoarthritis, or at least stop its progression, is by living in balance, as described in the lifestyle chapter.

17. POST-TRAUMATIC STRESS DISORDER

It has been estimated that 9% of the US population suffers from post-traumatic stress disorder sometime during their lives [68]. Women suffer from the condition more than men. Short-term memory loss, nightmares and flashbacks of traumatic events are common symptoms. Current therapy involves psychotherapy and antidepressants. Benzodiazepines can worsen the condition. Patients treat themselves with heroin, cocaine, amphetamine and marijuana [69].

CB1 receptors are elevated brain-wide in patients suffering from post-traumatic stress disorder [70]. At the same time, blood levels of anandamide and cortisol are low. This suggests that post-traumatic stress disorder is caused by excessive CB1 activity resulting in enhanced memory of traumatic events.

Marijuana smoking causes CB1 receptor downregulation [46] and may be useful in post-traumatic stress disorder. A recent clinical study found that patients who smoke marijuana (n=106) suffer less major depression and suicidal ideation than nonsmoking controls [68]. This backs up an earlier study where THC administered sublingually for 3 weeks to 10 patients decreased nightmares, anxiety and improved sleep quality [71]. Currently, the Canadian Agencies for Drugs and Technologies in Health recommend short term nabilone for patients suffering from nightmares.

CBD is an inhibitor of CB1 and may be able to cause the extinction of traumatic memories. A study of CBD in 11 patients found that 91% had improved symptoms in post-traumatic stress disorder [72]. CBD should be examined in clinical trials of post-traumatic stress disorder.

18. PSORIASIS

Psoriasis is caused by dysregulation of Th1 and Th17 cells that secrete interleukins, including IL-17A and IL-17F [73]. These interleukins induce inflammation and the secretion of chemokines that attract inflammatory cells into the skin. Several treatments are available, including antibodies that bind IL-17 and are reported to provide long-lasting relief, but not a cure.

Keratinocyte growth is regulated in part by endocannabinoids through CB1, CB2, PPARγ, and TRPV1 dependent mechanisms [74]. CBD, administered as a lotion, is a skin CB1 antagonist, a CB2 agonist, a TRPV1 activator/deactivator and was effective at improving symptoms in 5 psoriasis patients and needs to be tested in clinical trials [75].

19. TRAUMATIC BRAIN INJURY

Trauma to the brain causes damage to neurons and other cells. This damage involves oxidative stress, which can be decreased by glutathione. N-Acetyl-cysteine, a glutathione precursor, has been shown to improve symptoms in traumatic brain injury in a clinical trial [76]. Microglia become activated and migrate to the site of damage. These microglial cells are regulated by CB2 receptors and contain anandamide, 2-AG and the enzymes needed to make and degrade the endocannabinoids [77]. As neurons die, they are replaced by astrocytes that eventually form a glial scar. These astrocytes contain endocannabinoids, the enzymes to make and degrade endocannabinoids. These cellular changes in the brain may be why anandamide and 2-AG increase, cyclooxygenase-2 activity increases, as well as prostaglandins, leukotrienes, cytokines and chemokines. Blood vessels rupture and the blood-brain barrier becomes leaky in traumatic brain injury [77]. This leads to increased intracranial pressure and increased brain damage.

Smoking marijuana decreases CB1 receptor translation and endocannabinoid levels [46]. Several studies and meta-analyses have found that marijuana improves symptoms in traumatic brain injury and improves survival [78 - 80]. Cannabidiol decreases leakiness of the blood brain barrier, could be useful in traumatic brain injury, but has not been tested in clinical trials.

CONCLUSIONS

The balance necessary for good health depends on endocannabinoids and other eicosanoids. When this balance is endangered by improper lifestyles or disease, plant-based medicines can help. However, the complexity of the endocannabinoidome makes therapy difficult and sometimes unpredictable. The use of marijuana can provide effective therapy that may not last due to responses of the endocannabinoidome to therapy.

REFERENCES

[1]   Cristino L, Bisogno T, Di Marzo V. Cannabinoids and the expanded endocannabinoid system in neurological disorders. Nat Rev Neurol 2020; 16(1): 9-29.
        [http://dx.doi.org/10.1038/s41582-019-0284-z] [PMID: 31831863]

[2]   Lovinger D. Regulation of synaptic function by endocannabinoids. In Learning and Memory a Comprehensive Reference. New York: Elsevier 2009; 4: pp. 771-92.

[3]   Adams J, Parker K. Extracellular and Intracellular Signaling. London: Royal Society of Chemistry 2011.
        [http://dx.doi.org/10.1039/9781849733434]

[4]   Adams JD. The effects of yin, yang and qi in the skin on pain. Medicines (Basel) 2016; 3(1): 5.
        [http://dx.doi.org/10.3390/medicines3010005] [PMID: 28930115]

[5] Barbieri SS, Amadio P, Gianellini S, *et al.* Cyclooxygenase-2-derived prostacyclin regulates arterial thrombus formation by suppressing tissue factor in a sirtuin-1-dependent-manner. Circulation 2012; 126(11): 1373-84.
[http://dx.doi.org/10.1161/CIRCULATIONAHA.112.097295] [PMID: 22865892]

[6] Hinz B, Cheremina O, Brune K. Acetaminophen (paracetamol) is a selective cyclooxygenase-2 inhibitor in man. FASEB J 2008; 22(2): 383-90.
[http://dx.doi.org/10.1096/fj.07-8506com] [PMID: 17884974]

[7] Take Y, Koizumi S, Nagahisa A. Prostaglandin E receptor 4 antagonist in cancer immunotherapy: mechanisms of action. Front Immunol 2020; 11: 324.
[http://dx.doi.org/10.3389/fimmu.2020.00324] [PMID: 32210957]

[8] Brightling CE, Brusselle G, Altman P. The impact of the prostaglandin D_2 receptor 2 and its downstream effects on the pathophysiology of asthma. Allergy 2020; 75(4): 761-8.
[http://dx.doi.org/10.1111/all.14001] [PMID: 31355946]

[9] Adams J. Chronic pain can it be cured? J Pharmaceut Drug Devl 2017; 4: 105-9.

[10] Adams J. Chronic pain in the skin, sexual differences and neurogenic inflammation. J Altern Complement Integr Med 2019; 5: 073-5.
[http://dx.doi.org/10.24966/ACIM-7562/100073]

[11] Adams J. Chronic pain two cures. OBM Integ Comp Med 2018; 3
[http://dx.doi.org/10.21926/obm.icm.1804xxx]

[12] De Petrocellis L, Ligresti A, Moriello AS, *et al.* Effects of cannabinoids and cannabinoid-enriched Cannabis extracts on TRP channels and endocannabinoid metabolic enzymes. Br J Pharmacol 2011; 163(7): 1479-94.
[http://dx.doi.org/10.1111/j.1476-5381.2010.01166.x] [PMID: 21175579]

[13] Lutz B, Marsicano G, Maldonado R, Hillard CJ. The endocannabinoid system in guarding against fear, anxiety and stress. Nat Rev Neurosci 2015; 16(12): 705-18.
[http://dx.doi.org/10.1038/nrn4036] [PMID: 26585799]

[14] Mammen G, Rueda S, Roerecke M, Bonato S, Lev-Ran S, Rehm J. Association of Cannabis with long-term clinical symptoms in anxiety and mood disorders: A systematic review of prospective studies. J Clin Psychiat 2018.
[http://dx.doi.org/10.4088/JCP.17r11839]

[15] Mandolini GM, Lazzaretti M, Pigoni A, Oldani L, Delvecchio G, Brambilla P. Pharmacological properties of cannabidiol in the treatment of psychiatric disorders: a critical overview. Epidemiol Psychiatr Sci 2018; 27(4): 327-35.
[http://dx.doi.org/10.1017/S2045796018000239] [PMID: 29789034]

[16] Bauer AZ, Kriebel D. Prenatal and perinatal analgesic exposure and autism: an ecological link. Environ Health 2013; 12: 41.
[http://dx.doi.org/10.1186/1476-069X-12-41] [PMID: 23656698]

[17] Masarwa R, Levine H, Gorelik E, Reif S, Perlman A, Matok I. Prenatal exposure to acetaminophen and risk for attention deficit hyperactivity disorder and autistic spectrum disorder: A systematic review, meta-analysis, and meta-regression analysis of cohort studies. Am J Epidemiol 2018; 187(8): 1817-27.
[http://dx.doi.org/10.1093/aje/kwy086] [PMID: 29688261]

[18] Kerr DM, Downey L, Conboy M, Finn DP, Roche M. Alterations in the endocannabinoid system in the rat valproic acid model of autism. Behav Brain Res 2013; 249: 124-32.
[http://dx.doi.org/10.1016/j.bbr.2013.04.043] [PMID: 23643692]

[19] Yang F, Chen J, Miao MH, *et al.* Risk of autism spectrum disorder in offspring following paternal use of selective serotonin reuptake inhibitors before conception: a population-based cohort study. BMJ Open 2017; 7(12): e016368.

[http://dx.doi.org/10.1136/bmjopen-2017-016368] [PMID: 29275337]

[20]   Umathe SN, Manna SS, Jain NS. Involvement of endocannabinoids in antidepressant and anti-compulsive effect of fluoxetine in mice. Behav Brain Res 2011; 223(1): 125-34.
[http://dx.doi.org/10.1016/j.bbr.2011.04.031] [PMID: 21549765]

[21]   Brigida AL, Schultz S, Cascone M, Antonucci N, Siniscalco D. Endocannabinod signal dysregulation in autism spectrum disorders: A correlation link between inflammatory state and neuro-immune alterations. Int J Mol Sci 2017; 18(7): 1425.
[http://dx.doi.org/10.3390/ijms18071425] [PMID: 28671614]

[22]   Schultz S, Gould G. Acetaminophen use for fever in children associated with autism spectrum disorder. Autism Open Access 2016; 6(2): 170.
[http://dx.doi.org/10.4172/2165-7890.1000170]

[23]   Chen JA, Peñagarikano O, Belgard TG, Swarup V, Geschwind DH. The emerging picture of autism spectrum disorder: genetics and pathology. Annu Rev Pathol 2015; 10: 111-44.
[http://dx.doi.org/10.1146/annurev-pathol-012414-040405] [PMID: 25621659]

[24]   Korem N, Lange R, Hillard CJ, Akirav I. Role of beta-catenin and endocannabinoids in the nucleus accumbens in extinction in rats exposed to shock and reminders. Neuroscience 2017; 357: 285-94.
[http://dx.doi.org/10.1016/j.neuroscience.2017.06.015] [PMID: 28624572]

[25]   Azhari A, Azizan F, Esposito G. A systematic review of gut-immune-brain mechanisms in Autism Spectrum Disorder. Dev Psychobiol 2019; 61(5): 752-71.
[http://dx.doi.org/10.1002/dev.21803] [PMID: 30523646]

[26]   Bar-Lev Schleider L, Mechoulam R, Saban N, Meiri G, Novack V. Real life experience of medical Cannabis treatment in autism: Analysis of safety and efficacy. Sci Rep 2019; 9(1): 200-7.
[http://dx.doi.org/10.1038/s41598-018-37570-y] [PMID: 30655581]

[27]   Aran A, Cassuto H, Lubotzky A, Wattad N, Hazan E. Brief report: Cannabidiol-rich Cannabis in children with autism spectrum disorder and severe behavioral problems-a retrospective feasibility study. J Autism Dev Disord 2019; 49(3): 1284-8.
[http://dx.doi.org/10.1007/s10803-018-3808-2] [PMID: 30382443]

[28]   Benton-Gaillard J. Positive autism Intervention with cannabidiol: A case study. Am J Endocannabinoid Med 2019; 1: 56-9.

[29]   Fleury-Teixeira P, Caixeta FV, Ramires da Silva LC, Brasil-Neto JP, Malcher-Lopes R. Effects of CBD enriched Cannabis sativa extract on autism spectrum disorder symptoms an observational study of 18 participants undergoing compassionate use. Front Neurol 2019; 10: 1145.
[http://dx.doi.org/10.3389/fneur.2019.01145] [PMID: 31736860]

[30]   Aran A, Eylon M, Harel M, *et al.* Lower circulating endocannabinoid levels in children with autism spectrum disorder. 2019. Mol Autism
[http://dx.doi.org/10.1186/s13229-019-0256-6]

[31]   Couch DG, Cook H, Ortori C, Barrett D, Lund JN, O'Sullivan SE. Palmitoylethanolamide and cannabidiol prevent inflammation-induced hyperpermeability of the human gut *in vitro* and in vivo-a randomized, placebo-controlled, double-blind controlled trial. Inflamm Bowel Dis 2019; 25(6): 1006-18.
[http://dx.doi.org/10.1093/ibd/izz017] [PMID: 31054246]

[32]   Śledziński P, Zeyland J, Słomski R, Nowak A. The current state and future perspectives of cannabinoids in cancer biology. Cancer Med 2018; 7(3): 765-75.
[http://dx.doi.org/10.1002/cam4.1312] [PMID: 29473338]

[33]   Abrams DI, Guzman M. Cannabis in cancer care. Clin Pharmacol Ther 2015; 97(6): 575-86.
[http://dx.doi.org/10.1002/cpt.108] [PMID: 25777363]

[34]   Klimas NG, Salvato FR, Morgan R, Fletcher MA. Immunologic abnormalities in chronic fatigue syndrome. J Clin Microbiol 1990; 28(6): 1403-10.

[http://dx.doi.org/10.1128/jcm.28.6.1403-1410.1990] [PMID: 2166084]

[35]   Nakatomi Y, Mizuno K, Ishii A, *et al.* Neuroinflammation in patients with chronic fatigue syndrome/myalgic encephalomyelitis: An [11]C-(R)-PK11195 PET study. J Nucl Med 2014; 55(6): 945-50.
[http://dx.doi.org/10.2967/jnumed.113.131045] [PMID: 24665088]

[36]   Smith ME, Haney E, McDonagh M, *et al.* Treatment of myalgic encephalomyelitis/chronic fatigue syndrome: A systematic review for a national institutes of health pathways to prevention workshop. Ann Intern Med 2015; 162(12): 841-50.
[http://dx.doi.org/10.7326/M15-0114] [PMID: 26075755]

[37]   Fluge Ø, Rekeland IG, Lien K, *et al.* B-Lymphocyte depletion in patients with myalgic encephalomyelitis/chronic fatigue syndrome: A randomized, double-blind, placebo-controlled trial. Ann Intern Med 2019; 170(9): 585-93.
[http://dx.doi.org/10.7326/M18-1451] [PMID: 30934066]

[38]   Sarvaiya K, Goswami S. Investigation of the effects of vanilloids in chronic fatigue syndrome. Brain Res Bull 2016; 127: 187-94.
[http://dx.doi.org/10.1016/j.brainresbull.2016.09.015] [PMID: 27693335]

[39]   Calapai F, Cardia L, Sorbara EE, *et al.* Cannabinoids, blood–brain barrier, and brain disposition. Pharmaceutics 2020; 12(3): 265.
[http://dx.doi.org/10.3390/pharmaceutics12030265] [PMID: 32183416]

[40]   Gruden G, Barutta F, Kunos G, Pacher P. Role of the endocannabinoid system in diabetes and diabetic complications. Br J Pharmacol 2016; 173(7): 1116-27.
[http://dx.doi.org/10.1111/bph.13226] [PMID: 26076890]

[41]   Bermúdez-Silva FJ, Suárez J, Baixeras E, *et al.* Presence of functional cannabinoid receptors in human endocrine pancreas. Diabetologia 2008; 51(3): 476-87.
[http://dx.doi.org/10.1007/s00125-007-0890-y] [PMID: 18092149]

[42]   Horváth B, Mukhopadhyay P, Haskó G, Pacher P. The endocannabinoid system and plant-derived cannabinoids in diabetes and diabetic complications. Am J Pathol 2012; 180(2): 432-42.
[http://dx.doi.org/10.1016/j.ajpath.2011.11.003] [PMID: 22155112]

[43]   Penner EA, Buettner H, Mittleman MA. The impact of marijuana use on glucose, insulin, and insulin resistance among US adults. Am J Med 2013; 126(7): 583-9.
[http://dx.doi.org/10.1016/j.amjmed.2013.03.002] [PMID: 23684393]

[44]   Sidney S. Marijuana use and type 2 diabetes mellitus: a review. Curr Diab Rep 2016; 16(11): 117.
[http://dx.doi.org/10.1007/s11892-016-0795-6] [PMID: 27747490]

[45]   Danielsson AK, Lundin A, Yaregal A, Östenson CG, Allebeck P, Agardh EE. Cannabis use as risk or protection for type 2 diabetes: A longitudinal study of 18 000 Swedish men and women. J Diabetes Res 2016; 2016: 6278709.
[http://dx.doi.org/10.1155/2016/6278709] [PMID: 27843955]

[46]   D'Souza DC, Cortes-Briones JA, Ranganathan M, *et al.* Rapid changes in cannabinoid 1 receptor availability in cannabis-dependent male subjects after abstinence from Cannabis. Biol Psychiatry Cogn Neurosci Neuroimaging 2016; 1(1): 60-7.
[http://dx.doi.org/10.1016/j.bpsc.2015.09.008] [PMID: 29560896]

[47]   Sugaya Y, Kano M. Control of excessive neural circuit excitability and prevention of epileptic seizures by endocannabinoid signaling. Cell Mol Life Sci 2018; 75(15): 2793-811.
[http://dx.doi.org/10.1007/s00018-018-2834-8] [PMID: 29737364]

[48]   Seidelmann SB, Claggett B, Cheng S, *et al.* Dietary carbohydrate intake and mortality: a prospective cohort study and meta-analysis. Lancet Public Health 2018; 3(9): e419-28.
[http://dx.doi.org/10.1016/S2468-2667(18)30135-X] [PMID: 30122560]

[49]   Fung TT, van Dam RM, Hankinson SE, Stampfer M, Willett WC, Hu FB. Low-carbohydrate diets and

all-cause and cause-specific mortality: two cohort studies. Ann Intern Med 2010; 153(5): 289-98.
[http://dx.doi.org/10.7326/0003-4819-153-5-201009070-00003] [PMID: 20820038]

[50] Bari M, Rapino C, Mozetic P, Maccarone M. The endocannabinoid system in gp120-mediated insults and HIV-associated dementia. Exp Neurol 2010; 224(1): 74-84.
[http://dx.doi.org/10.1016/j.expneurol.2010.03.025] [PMID: 20353779]

[51] Xu C, Hermes DJ, Nwanguma B, *et al.* Endocannabinoids exert CB_1 receptor-mediated neuroprotective effects in models of neuronal damage induced by HIV-1 Tat protein. Mol Cell Neurosci 2017; 83: 92-102.
[http://dx.doi.org/10.1016/j.mcn.2017.07.003] [PMID: 28733129]

[52] Lutge EE, Gray A, Siegfried N. The medical use of cannabis for reducing morbidity and mortality in patients with HIV/AIDS. Cochrane Database Syst Rev 2013; (4): CD005175.
[http://dx.doi.org/10.1002/14651858.CD005175.pub3] [PMID: 23633327]

[53] Hasenoehrl C, Taschler U, Storr M, Schicho R. The gastrointestinal tract - a central organ of cannabinoid signaling in health and disease. Neurogastroenterol Motil 2016; 28(12): 1765-80.
[http://dx.doi.org/10.1111/nmo.12931] [PMID: 27561826]

[54] Russo EB. Clinical endocannabinoid deficiency reconsidered: Current research supports the theory in migraine, fibromyalgia, irritable Bowel, and other treatment-resistant syndromes. Cannabis Cannabinoid Res 2016; 1(1): 154-65.
[http://dx.doi.org/10.1089/can.2016.0009] [PMID: 28861491]

[55] Goyal H, Singla U, Gupta U, May E. Role of cannabis in digestive disorders. Eur J Gastroenterol Hepatol 2017; 29(2): 135-43.
[http://dx.doi.org/10.1097/MEG.0000000000000779] [PMID: 27792038]

[56] Martínez V, Iriondo De-Hond A, Borrelli F, Capasso R, Del Castillo MD, Abalo R. Cannabidiol and other non-psychoactive cannabinoids for prevention and treatment of gastrointestinal disorders: Useful nutraceuticals? Int J Mol Sci 2020; 21(9): 3067.
[http://dx.doi.org/10.3390/ijms21093067] [PMID: 32357565]

[57] Olesen J, Burstein R, Ashina M, Tfelt-Hansen P. Origin of pain in migraine: evidence for peripheral sensitisation. Lancet Neurol 2009; 8(7): 679-90.
[http://dx.doi.org/10.1016/S1474-4422(09)70090-0] [PMID: 19539239]

[58] Pan Y, Chen F, Huang S, *et al.* TRPA1 and TRPM8 receptors may promote local vasodilation that aggravates oxaliplatin-induced peripheral neuropathy amenable to 17β-estradiol treatment. Curr Neurovasc Res 2016; 13(4): 309-17.
[http://dx.doi.org/10.2174/1567202613666160601144254] [PMID: 27262300]

[59] Rhyne DN, Anderson SL, Gedde M, Borgelt LM. Effects of medical marijuana on migraine headache frequency in an adult population. Pharmacotherapy 2016; 36(5): 505-10.
[http://dx.doi.org/10.1002/phar.1673] [PMID: 26749285]

[60] Yamamoto T, Mulpuri Y, Izraylev M, *et al.* Selective targeting of peripheral cannabinoid receptors prevents behavioral symptoms and sensitization of trigeminal neurons in mouse models of migraine and medication overuse headache. Pain 2021; 162(8): 2246-62.
[http://dx.doi.org/10.1097/j.pain.0000000000002214] [PMID: 33534356]

[61] Zajicek J, Ball S, Wright D, *et al.* Effect of dronabinol on progression in progressive multiple sclerosis (CUPID): a randomised, placebo-controlled trial. Lancet Neurol 2013; 12(9): 857-65.
[http://dx.doi.org/10.1016/S1474-4422(13)70159-5] [PMID: 23856559]

[62] Zajicek JP, Hobart JC, Slade A, Barnes D, Mattison PG. Multiple sclerosis and extract of cannabis: results of the MUSEC trial. J Neurol Neurosurg Psychiatry 2012; 83(11): 1125-32.
[http://dx.doi.org/10.1136/jnnp-2012-302468] [PMID: 22791906]

[63] Novotna A, Mares J, Ratcliffe S, *et al.* A randomized, double-blind, placebo-controlled, parallel-group, enriched-design study of nabiximols* (Sativex®), as add-on therapy, in subjects with refractory

spasticity caused by multiple sclerosis. Eur J Neurol 2011; 18(9): 1122-31.
[http://dx.doi.org/10.1111/j.1468-1331.2010.03328.x] [PMID: 21362108]

[64]   Katz-Talmor D, Katz I, Porat-Katz BS, Shoenfeld Y. Cannabinoids for the treatment of rheumatic diseases - where do we stand? Nat Rev Rheumatol 2018; 14(8): 488-98.
[http://dx.doi.org/10.1038/s41584-018-0025-5] [PMID: 29884803]

[65]   Dunn S, Wilkinson J, Crawford A, Bunning R, Le Maitre C. Expression of cannabinoid receptors in human osteoarthritic cartilage: implications for future therapies. Cannabis Cannabinoid Res 2016; 1(1): 3-15.
[http://dx.doi.org/10.1089/can.2015.0001]

[66]   Barrie N, Kuruppu V, Manolios E, Ali M, Moghaddam M, Manolios N. Endocannabinoids in arthritis: current views and perspective. Int J Rheum Dis 2017; 20(7): 789-97.
[http://dx.doi.org/10.1111/1756-185X.13146] [PMID: 28736968]

[67]   Berg MVD, John M, Black M, *et al.* Cannabis-based medicinal products in arthritis, a painful conundrum. N Z Med J 2020; 133(1515): 35-45.
[PMID: 32438375]

[68]   Lake S, Kerr T, Buxton J, *et al.* Does cannabis use modify the effect of post-traumatic stress disorder on severe depression and suicidal ideation? Evidence from a population-based cross-sectional study of Canadians. J Psychopharmacol 2020; 34(2): 181-8.journals.sagepub.com/home/jop
[http://dx.doi.org/10.1177/0269881119882806] [PMID: 31684805]

[69]   Bonn-Miller   M,   Rousseau   G.   Marijuana   yse   and   PTSD   among   veterans.
https://www.ptsd.va.gov/professional/treat/cooccurring/marijuana_ptsd_vets.asp

[70]   Neumeister A, Normandin MD, Pietrzak RH, *et al.* Elevated brain cannabinoid CB1 receptor availability in post-traumatic stress disorder: a positron emission tomography study. Mol Psychiatry 2013; 18(9): 1034-40.
[http://dx.doi.org/10.1038/mp.2013.61] [PMID: 23670490]

[71]   Roitman P, Mechoulam R, Cooper-Kazaz R, Shalev A. Preliminary, open-label, pilot study of add-on oral Δ9-tetrahydrocannabinol in chronic post-traumatic stress disorder. Clin Drug Investig 2014; 34(8): 587-91.
[http://dx.doi.org/10.1007/s40261-014-0212-3] [PMID: 24935052]

[72]   Elms L, Shannon S, Hughes S, Lewis N. Cannabidiol in the treatment of post-traumatic stress disorder: A case series. J Altern Complement Med 2019; 25(4): 392-7.
[http://dx.doi.org/10.1089/acm.2018.0437] [PMID: 30543451]

[73]   Diani M, Altomare G, Reali E. Helper cell subsets in clinical manifestations of psoriasis. J Immunol Res 2016; 2016: 7692024.
[http://dx.doi.org/10.1155/2016/7692024] [PMID: 27595115]

[74]   Río CD, Millán E, García V, Appendino G, DeMesa J, Muñoz E. The endocannabinoid system of the skin. A potential approach for the treatment of skin disorders. Biochem Pharmacol 2018; 157: 122-33.
[http://dx.doi.org/10.1016/j.bcp.2018.08.022] [PMID: 30138623]

[75]   Palmieri B, Laurino C, Vadalà M. A therapeutic effect of cbd-enriched ointment in inflammatory skin diseases and cutaneous scars. Clin Ther 2019; 170(2): e93-9.
[http://dx.doi.org/10.7417/CT.2019.2116] [PMID: 30993303]

[76]   Hoffer ME, Balaban C, Slade MD, Tsao JW, Hoffer B. Amelioration of acute sequelae of blast induced mild traumatic brain injury by N-acetyl cysteine: a double-blind, placebo controlled study. PLoS One 2013; 8(1): e54163.
[http://dx.doi.org/10.1371/journal.pone.0054163] [PMID: 23372680]

[77]   Schurman LD, Lichtman AH. Endocannabinoids: A promising impact for traumatic brain injury. Front Pharmacol 2017; 8: 69.
[http://dx.doi.org/10.3389/fphar.2017.00069] [PMID: 28261100]

[78]   Nguyen BM, Kim D, Bricker S, *et al.* Effect of marijuana use on outcomes in traumatic brain injury. Am Surg 2014; 80(10): 979-83.
[http://dx.doi.org/10.1177/000313481408001015] [PMID: 25264643]

[79]   Hindocha C, Cousijn J, Rall M, Bloomfield MAP. The effectiveness of cannabinoids in the treatment of posttraumatic stress disorder (PTSD): A systematic review. J Dual Diagn 2020; 16(1): 120-39.
[http://dx.doi.org/10.1080/15504263.2019.1652380] [PMID: 31479625]

[80]   Orsolini L, Chiappini S, Volpe U, *et al.* Use of medicinal Cannabis and synthetic cannabinoids in post-traumatic stress disorder (PTSD): A systematic review. Medicina (Kaunas) 2019; 55(9): 525.
[http://dx.doi.org/10.3390/medicina55090525] [PMID: 31450833]

CHAPTER 6

The Antioxidant System and Balance

Abstract: The body is protected by glutathione, the most important antioxidant. Glutathione protects the body from oxidative stress, hydrogen peroxide toxicity and lipid peroxidation. Patients seek dietary antioxidants to help with their health. Lifestyle changes such as daily exercise and getting rid of excess weight help maintain glutathione and health.

Keywords: Antioxidants, Catalase, Gamma-glutamyl transferase, – Glutaredoxin, Glutathione peroxidase, Glutathione, Hydrogen peroxide, Isoprostane, Peroxiredoxin, Pyroglutamate, Vitamin E.

1. INTRODUCTION

The body depends on antioxidants for protection against reactive oxygen species and other reactive species that derive from the fact that humans breathe air. Air is processed in the mitochondrial oxidative phosphorylation system to make ATP. A side product of this respiratory system is the generation of reactive oxygen species such as superoxide radical anion that interacts with superoxide dismutase or manganese superoxide dismutase to form hydrogen peroxide. Oxygen radicals produced by this system are short-lived and do not usually cross mitochondrial and other membranes. It has been estimated that 0.1-2% of the oxygen used by mitochondria makes a superoxide radical anion [1]. Hydrogen peroxide crosses membranes due to channels called peroxiporins and is a powerful oxidant that within minutes damages DNA and other macromolecules [2]. The body detoxifies hydrogen peroxide through the actions of peroxiredoxins, glutathione peroxidase and catalase.

2. HYDROGEN PEROXIDE SIGNALING

Hydrogen peroxide transmits signals from one organelle to another since it crosses membranes at peroxiporin pores. It readily penetrates into the nucleus, damages DNA and activates poly(ADP-ribose) polymerase [3, 4]. Poly(ADP-ribose) polymerase upregulates the transcriptional activity of nuclear factor erythroid 2 related factors 2 (Nrf2) and enhances the interaction between antioxidant response elements (ARE), Nrf2 and MafG [5]. Nrf2 is a transcription factor that is involved in the regulation of redox homeostasis, such as during oxidative stress. It is normally found in the cytosol but is translocated into the nucleus during oxidative stress, where it is stabilized by heterodimerization with small Maf proteins, such as MafG. Poly(ADP-ribose) polymerase binds to ARE and NafG, which enhances the ability of Nrf2 to bind to ARE and MafG. This increases the transcription of Nrf2 target genes. These genes include glutathione transferase, NADPH dehydrogenase (quinone 1), glutamate-cysteine ligase, sulfiredoxin 1, thioredoxin reductase 1, heme oxygenase 1, UDP glucuronosyltransferase, and multidrug resistance-associated proteins.

P53 is stabilized by cytosolic NADPH dehydrogenase (quinone 1) [6], and is involved in the regulation of DNA repair genes. The progression of apoptosis is controlled by P53. This is involved in hydrogen peroxide induction of a number of apoptosis-inducing and inhibiting proteins [7].

Hydrogen peroxide also oxidizes sulfur, such as in cysteine to sulfenic (SOH), sulfinic (SO_2H), and sulfonic (SO_3H) acids [8]. It promotes the formation of disulfides between proteins and glutathione. Nrf2 is normally deactivated following ubiquitination by Kelch-like ECH-associated protein 1 (KEAP1). This leads to proteasomal degradation. Hydrogen peroxide oxidizes Cys151, Cys171, Cys273, Cys288 of KEAP1, which decreases its activity and inhibits its ability to deactivate Nrf2. Several other protein cysteines are oxidized by hydrogen peroxide leading to changes in activity, including forkhead box O3 transcription factor, NFkB subunits and tumor suppressor phosphatase (PTEN).

3. CATALASE

Catalase is a heme enzyme found in peroxisomes (Fig. **1**) that can change millions of molecules of hydrogen peroxide into water and oxygen every second [9]. Catalase also uses hydrogen peroxide to oxidize ethanol, formaldehyde, formic acid, phenols, acetaldehyde and other compounds. NADPH is tightly bound to catalase and is involved in hydride transfer that prevents the deactivation of catalase and accumulation of compound II, the inactive form of catalase [10]. Humans born with little catalase activity, acatalasemia usually have normal health.

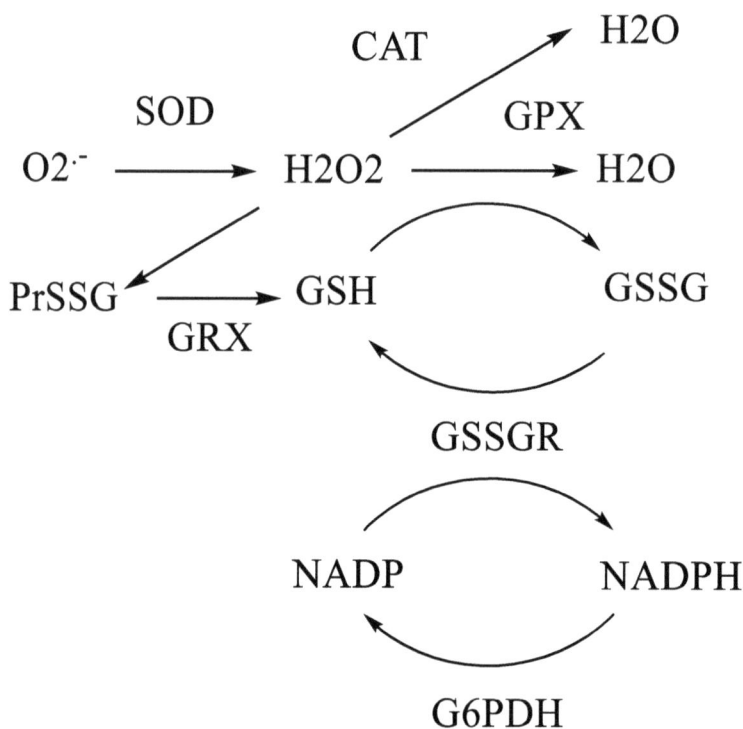

Fig. (1). The glutathione antioxidant system. Glutathione (GSH) and glutathione disulfide (GSSG) interact with hydrogen peroxide formed by superoxide dismutase (SOD). Glutathione peroxidase (GPX) catalyzes the detoxification of hydrogen peroxide. Glutathione disulfide reductase (GSSGR) maintains the glutathione redox state at the expense of NADPH. NADP is reduced by glucose-6-phosphate dehydrogenase. Catalase also detoxifies hydrogen peroxide. Hydrogen peroxide oxidizes protein figuresulfhydryls forming glutathione-protein mixed disulfides (PRSSG).

Peroxisomes are found in every cell in the body and are involved in hydrogen peroxide detoxification, very long-chain fatty acid catabolism, branched-chain fatty acid catabolism, production of plasmalogens and other functions [8]. Plasmalogens are ether phospholipids that are important in the membranes of heart and brain cells, especially myelin [11].

4. GLUTATHIONE

Glutathione is a tripeptide, γ-glutamyl-cysteinyl glycine, and is the most important antioxidant in the body. It is synthesized in the cytoplasms of every cell due to the actions of glutamate-cysteine ligase and glutathione synthetase. Glutamate cysteine ligase makes γ-glutamylcysteine at the expense of ATP. Glutathione synthetase adds glycine to this at the expense of ATP. Glutamate cysteine ligase is the rate-limiting enzyme in glutathione synthesis and is regulated by oxidative stress, glutathione depletion, Nrf2, AP-1 and NFkB signaling [12]. Glutathione synthetase deficiency is a rare condition that causes a number of birth defects, including hemolytic anemia, metabolic acidosis and neurological defects.

Quantitating glutathione and glutathione disulfide is not an easy matter. Glutathione oxidizes quickly during tissue homogenization and extraction [13]. Stabilization of glutathione by reaction with N-ethylmaleimide or a similar derivatizing reagent can solve this problem. In addition, glutathione is rapidly degraded by γ-glutamyl transferase in human plasma and cellular homogenates [14]. This can be prevented by acidification or filtration to remove the protein [13, 15]. Tissue levels of glutathione are typically more than 200 fold higher than levels of glutathione disulfide [13].

Glutathione is released from the liver into the plasma [16] and may serve as a cysteine source for other organs such as during times of food deprivation. Glutathione disulfide is released from the liver, lungs and other organs during oxidative stress [13, 17]. Multidrug resistance-associated proteins are the channels that release intracellular glutathione disulfide into the plasma [14]. This may be how the liver and other organs maintain intracellular redox balance. It is also possible that plasma glutathione disulfide is an extracellular signal to other organs that oxidative stress-inducing toxic compounds have been introduced into the body. This is further described in the γ-glutamyl transferase and pyroglutamate sections. Glutathione disulfide can be sequestered in vacuoles and endoplasmic reticula by some organs [18]. The brain retains glutathione disulfide during oxidative stress [19]. It is not known if brain glutathione disulfide is sequestered in vacuoles. This sequestration may be how some organs maintain intracellular redox balance.

The glutathione redox state can be expressed by the electrochemical reduction potential, which is usually about -0.24 V [20]. The reduction potential for NADP/NADPH is -0.32 V. This indicates that NADPH can reduce glutathione disulfide, such as due to the actions of glutathione disulfide reductase. During severe oxidative stress in the brain, such as from tert-butylhydroperoxide, the GSSG/GSH reduction potential decreases to -0.15 V [20], while the NADP/NADPH reduction potential decreases to -0.3 V. During severe oxidative stress, NADPH can still reduce glutathione disulfide.

In cell culture, the reduction potential of GSSG/GSH can be -0.32 V [18]. It has been reported that when the reduction potential of GSSG/GSH increases to -0.17 V, apoptosis may occur [21]. In the brain subjected to tert-butyl hydroperoxide oxidative stress, both apoptosis and necrosis were observed [22, 23]. Glutathione depletion increases the reduction potential and seems to be involved in other forms of cell death, including necroptosis, ferroptosis and autophagy [24].

Glutathione is required for DNA synthesis, immune system function, the formation of leukotrienes and the detoxification of some drugs and other xenobiotics [25]. Several enzymes require glutathione as a cofactor or substrate, including glyoxalase, leukotriene C4 synthase, prostaglandin-endoperoxide synthase and prostaglandin E synthase [25]. Glyoxalase removes toxic aldehydes from the cell and prevents advanced glycation end-product formation, which may be involved in aging. Glutathione depletion, such as during aging, may decrease the activity of glyoxalase and increase the formation of advanced glycation end products.

There are a number of ways to ensure proper glutathione synthesis in the body. N-Acetylcysteine has been used for many years to increase glutathione synthesis, such as during glutathione depletion by acetaminophen. The Mediterranean diet or a diet including asparagus, avocado, cucumber, green beans and spinach, supports glutathione synthesis [26]. Exercise increases cellular glutathione levels and decreases glutathione disulfide levels [27]. This is contrary to what some may expect. Exercise increases oxygen use, may increase hydrogen peroxide production, and decrease glutathione due to the actions of glutathione peroxidase. The fact is that regular exercise increases glutathione and decreases glutathione disulfide.

5. GLUTATHIONYLATION

The addition of glutathione to an enzyme changes a protein sulfhydryl to a disulfide, adds a negative charge to the protein and adds bulky glutathione. This alters protein conformation and possibly activity. Proteins that have altered activity after the formation of protein glutathione mixed disulfides include cytoskeletal proteins, calcium homeostasis proteins, energy metabolism proteins, signaling pathway proteins, antioxidant enzymes and protein folding enzymes [28]. Glutathionylation occurs spontaneously and can be catalyzed by glutathione transferase pi. The cell signaling proteins JNK, c-jun and TRAF2 are glutathionylated by glutathione transferase pi resulting in loss of activity [28].

Several enzymes are glutathionylated as a regulatory measure during oxidative stress. Protein kinase A loses activity upon glutathionylation [28]. The phosphatidylinositol 3-kinase Akt p53 pathway is regulated by glutathionylation [28]. PTEN is reversibly deactivated by glutathionylation, as is Ser/Thr protein phosphatase 2A. These enzymes regulate Akt and its pathway. Glutathionylation of p53 inhibits its ability to recognize its DNA binding sites.

IkB phosphorylation by IkB kinase is inhibited by glutathionylation of Cys179 [28]. NFkB DNA binding is inhibited by glutathionylation at Cys62. Glutathionylation of c-Jun causes it to lose activity, which is also true of MAP/ERK kinase 1. Peroxiredoxins are glutathionylated at the active site cysteine with loss of activity.

Fas receptor is inhibited by glutathionylation, which inhibits apoptosis [28]. Caspases are also involved in apoptosis. Caspase 3 is inhibited by glutathionylation.

Sarcoplasmic endoplasmic reticulum calcium ATPase (SERCA) transports calcium into the sarcoplasmic reticulum, which decreases potentially toxic levels of calcium in the cytosol [28]. Glutathionylation of SERCA activates the calcium uptake system.

Proteasomal protein degradation involves ubiquitination of proteins followed by proteolysis. The 20S core particle of the proteasome complex is regulated by glutathionylation [28].

Protein folding occurs in the endoplasmic reticula, where an oxidizing environment allows protein disulfide formation and other events that are required for normal protein folding. During stress to the endoplasmic reticulum, misfolded proteins accumulate, which stimulates the unfolded protein response. Various kinases are involved in this response, including JNK, which is regulated by glutathionylation [28]. Chaperone proteins, such as protein disulfide isomerase, are involved in the unfolded protein response. Protein disulfide isomerase is subject to glutathionylation [28].

Serpins are proteases that are important in the bone marrow. Serpin A1 inhibits neutrophil elastase [28]. Serpin A3 inhibits cathepsin G. Both enzymes are regulated by glutathionylation.

6. GLUTATHIONE PEROXIDASE

The major means of hydrogen peroxide detoxification is cytosolic glutathione peroxidase (Fig. **1**). It is more efficient than catalase at deactivating hydrogen peroxide [29]. It is found in all cells in all compartments. The enzyme contains selenocysteine and is active due to the formation of the anion of selenocysteine. Low dietary intake of selenium correlates with increased cancer incidence [29]. There are several forms of glutathione peroxidase, with glutathione peroxidase 1 being the most abundant and most catalytically important in terms of hydrogen peroxide deactivation. The hydrogen peroxide is reduced to water at the expense of glutathione which is oxidized to glutathione disulfide. Glutathione disulfide reductase then reduces glutathione disulfide back to glutathione at the expense of NADPH. Therefore, hydrogen peroxide signaling, glutathione signaling and NADPH signaling pathways are all connected through glutathione peroxidase 1.

Oxygen tension regulates the transcription of glutathione peroxidase through oxygen response elements [29]. Hypoxia increases the activity of oxygen response element proteins. Glutathione peroxidase transcription is also regulated by NFkB and activator protein-1 [29]. Nitric oxide, peroxynitrite and other reactive species deactivate glutathione peroxidase. Phosphorylation by tyrosine kinases such as Arg and c-Abl, activates glutathione peroxidase.

Glutathione peroxidase 4 deactivates lipid hydroperoxides, cholesterol hydroperoxides and is involved in the synthesis of eicosanoids [30]. The enzyme reduces the hydroperoxides of 5-hydroperoxy-eicosatetraenoic acid (5-HpETE), 12-HpETE, and 15-HpETE as well as other lipid hydroperoxides to lipid hydroxyl forms (Fig. **2**) [31]. Glutathione peroxidase 4 regulates apoptosis and ferroptosis [30]. Glutathione depletion due to excess glutathione peroxidase 4 activity leads to decreased activity of glutathione peroxidase 4. As this activity decreases, lipid hydroperoxides increase. Ferroptosis is caused by the excess formation of lipid hydroperoxides resulting in the release of iron from cellular ferritin. Free iron, also called labile iron, in the cell, causes lipid peroxidation leading to ferroptosis, which is a form of programmed cell death. Ferroptosis is an uncommon form of cell death.

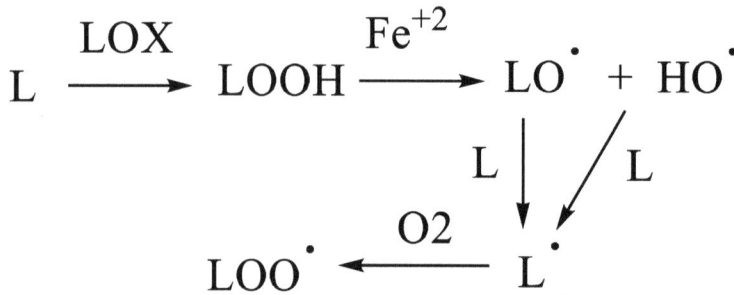

$$L \xrightarrow{\text{LOX}} LOOH \xrightarrow{\text{Fe}^{+2}} LO^{\bullet} + HO^{\bullet}$$

$$LOO^{\bullet} \xleftarrow{\text{O2}} L^{\bullet}$$

Fig. (2). Lipid peroxidation of arachidonic acid and linolenic acid is catalyzed by12/15 lipoxygenase (LOX) that forms lipid hydroperoxides of membrane bound lipids. Labile iron cleaves these hydroperoxides to release hydroxyl radical and lipoxyl radical (LO·). These radicals abstract hydrogens for neighboring lipids to form lipid radicals (L·) that are oxidized by oxygen to form lipid peroxyl radicals (LOO·).

7. GLUTAREDOXIN/THIOREDOXIN

Glutaredoxin is found in the nucleus, mitochondria, and cytoplasms of all cells

[32]. It is involved in glutathione redox signaling, iron-sulfur cluster biosynthesis, and iron sensing. Hydrogen peroxide oxidizes protein thiols to form sulfenic acids that react with glutathione to form protein-glutathione mixed disulfides [33]. These mixed disulfides may change the conformation of a protein and alter its activity. Glutaredoxin and thioredoxin reduce protein glutathione mixed disulfides back to the original sulfide and restore enzymatic activity. Glutaredoxin uses glutathione as a reducing agent to release glutathione form mixed disulfides. As a consequence, glutathione disulfide is produced by glutaredoxin. Thioredoxin also reduces protein glutathione mixed disulfides to release glutathione and restore the original protein. Thioredoxin is then reduced by NADPH due to the actions of thioredoxin reductase.

This is the basis of hydrogen peroxide signaling of oxidative stress from organelle to organelle inside the cell. As protein sulfenic acids are formed by hydrogen peroxide, glutathione spontaneously reacts to form mixed disulfides that alter enzyme activity. This signals the occurrence of oxidative stress. As the cell recovers from oxidative stress, glutaredoxin and thioredoxin restore enzyme activity.

Glutaredoxin usually catalyzes the release of glutathione from proteins. It can also catalyze the glutathionylation of some proteins, including glyceraldehyde 3-phosphate dehydrogenase, actin, and protein tyrosine phosphatase 1B [28].

8. PEROXIREDOXIN

Peroxiredoxins are found in every cell and reduce both hydrogen peroxide and peroxynitrite [34]. They are critical to hydrogen peroxide signaling. At low hydrogen peroxide levels, peroxiredoxins reduce hydrogen peroxide to water. However, during oxidative stress, when hydrogen peroxide production is high, hydrogen peroxide deactivates peroxiredoxins. This allows hydrogen peroxide to signal that oxidative stress is in progress. As oxidative stress is resolved, peroxiredoxin activity is restored. This occurs due to the activity of sulfiredoxin that reduces peroxiredoxin, restoring activity [34].

9. GAMMA-GLUTAMYL TRANSFERASE

G-Glutamyl transferase is involved in rescuing cysteine from plasma glutathione and cystine from plasma glutathione disulfide [14]. Glutamate is released by the enzyme as well (Fig. **3**). The enzyme is bound to the extracellular membranes of cells in the kidney, brain, bile duct, pancreas, heart, and seminal vesicles. The cysteine released is transported into cells by alanine, serine, cysteine transporters.

Cystine is taken up into cells by the xc- cystine/glutamate antiporter. G-Glutamyl transferase releases glutamate and cysteinyl glycine from glutathione. Cysteinylglycine is cleaved to the individual amino acids by dipeptidases.

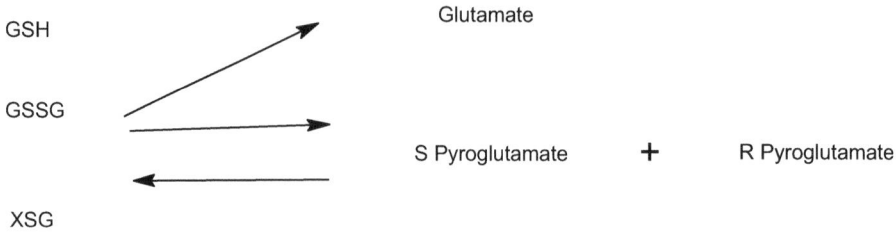

Fig. (3). Glutathione(GSH), glutathione disulfide (GSSG) and glutathione adducts of xenobiotics (XSG) release glutamic acid in the plasma due to the actions of γ-glutamyl transferase. Alternatively, glutathione, glutathione disulfide or glutathione adducts of xenobiotics produce pyroglutamic acid due to the actions of γ-glutamyl cyclotransferase. Pyroglutamate is converted to glutamate by 5-oxoprolinase at the expense of ATP.

Another function of γ-glutamyl transferase is to form mercapturic acids from glutathione adducts of toxic xenobiotics [14]. Glutamate is released by the enzyme and the cysteinyl glycine adduct of the xenobiotic. A peptidase cleaves glycine from this making the cysteine adduct of the xenobiotic. N-Acetyltransferase acetylates this to make the mercapturic acid that is lost in the urine. Xenobiotics that form glutathione adducts can be responsible for the depletion of cellular glutathione.

The expression of γ-glutamyl transferase on tumor cells allows the cells to capture cysteine and synthesize glutathione. These cells are drug-resistant. Tumors with high γ-glutamyl transferase activity are associated with poor survival [35].

Increased serum γ-glutamyl transferase activity is associated with poor prognosis in several diseases [36], such as alcohol-related liver disease, metabolic syndrome, coronary heart disease, and heart failure. These are diseases caused by poor lifestyles and diet. It is not clear how γ-glutamyl transferase is released from cell membranes into the plasma.

It has been proposed the serum γ-glutamyl transferase activity indicates the depletion of cellular glutathione, such as by toxic xenobiotics [36]. It is also possible that serum γ-glutamyl transferase activity is an indication of the release of iron from damaged red blood cells or plasma ferritin. G-Glutamyl transferase can be a pro-oxidant enzyme in the presence of labile iron. Increased serum ferritin is predictive of poor prognosis in several diseases, although it is not as good a predictor as serum γ-glutamyl transferase activity.

10. PYROGLUTAMATE

Glutamate is a degradation product of plasma glutathione, glutathione disulfide and glutathione adducts of xenobiotics due to the actions of γ-glutamyl transferase. Glutamate is cyclized by γ-glutamyl acyltransferase to form a lactam derivative called pyroglutamate or 5-oxoproline (Fig. **3**). Pyroglutamate is converted to glutamate by 5-oxoprolinase [37]. This appears to be a detoxification pathway. Congestive heart failure patients with high plasma levels of pyroglutamate have a worse clinical prognosis. Burn patients have high plasma and urinary levels of pyroglutamate [38]. This demonstrates the importance of the skin in glutathione regulation in the body. It is not known how pyroglutamate influences disease prognosis or the glutathione pathway.

11. ISOPROSTANES

Isoprostanes are nonclassical eicosanoids formed by free radical peroxidation of lipids [39]. This does not involve cyclooxygenase or lipoxygenase (Fig. **4**). Plasma and urinary isoprostanes are considered biomarkers of lipid peroxidation induced by oxidative stress. The most prevalent isoprostanes are the F2-isoprostanes that are produced from arachidonic acid. Isoprostanes are hyperalgesic when applied to skin sensory neurons [40]. They also increase the release of inflammatory neurokinins from skin sensory neurons. These neurokinins travel in the blood to sites of inflammation and increase the inflammation. This makes isoprostanes inflammatory agents and pain-producing agents. One of the inflammatory actions of F2-isoprostanes is the induction of neutrophil adhesion which is involved in atherosclerosis [41].

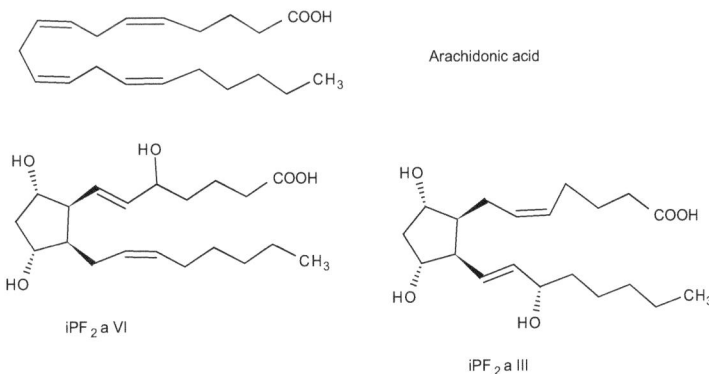

Fig. (4). Two isoprostanes iPF2a-VI and iPF2a-III, made from arachidonic acid by oxygen free radicals.

Cigarette smoking increases plasma and urinary isoprostane levels [42], indicating that smoking induces oxidative stress in the lungs and possibly other organs. Asthma is an inflammatory condition that involves isoprostane production in the lungs and exhalation in the breath. Acupuncture improves asthma control and decreases breath isoprostane production [43]. Systemic sclerosis appears to involve oxidative stress and isoprostane production [44]. Age related macular degeneration involves inflammation of the retina, especially in diabetes. Urinary F2-isoprostanes increase in age related macular degeneration [45].

Acute exercise increases plasma and muscle F2-isoprostane levels for a while [46]. This may be due to oxidative stress induced by physical exertion, which the body adapts to. Chronic exercise, such as daily exercise for several weeks, tends to decrease urinary F2-isoprostane levels. The body appears to adapt to the oxidative stress induced by daily exercise, becomes stronger and healthier.

12. VITAMIN E

Cell culture studies and laboratory animal experiments have indicated for many years that vitamin E inhibits lipid peroxidation by stopping free radical propagation. Vitamin E supplementation up to 1200 mg daily for 3 weeks had no effect on isoprostane production in smokers [47]. A study of the effects of vitamin E in patients with polygenic hypercholesterolemia found that vitamin E doses of 1600 or 3200 mg for 20 weeks decreased plasma isoprostane levels [48]. Overweight patients with body mass indices above 27 kg/m2 were administered 1200 mg daily of vitamin E for 3 months. Plasma isoprostane levels decreased in these patients [49].

These results indicate that very high dose vitamin E may have an effect on lipid peroxidation in patients. There was no assessment of vitamin E toxicity in these patients. Vitamin E has been reported in several clinical trials to increase or not decrease the risk of death from heart disease. It may be better for patients to improve their lifestyles and get rid of excess weight rather than taking high doses of vitamin E for months.

13. ANTIOXIDANTS

It is critical to keep in mind that antioxidants cannot make up for a toxic lifestyle. Patients must be encouraged to stop their toxic lifestyles and live in balance. Eating a balanced diet, as discussed in the lifestyles chapter, provides all the antioxidants needed from fruit and vegetables. People who eat too much meat and not enough fruit and vegetables must be encouraged to eat balanced diets.

Antioxidants cannot alter the need to eat fruit and vegetables. Adding fruit and vegetable-derived antioxidants to the diet is expensive and may provide supplements that are not as well absorbed from the gut as antioxidants eaten in fruits and vegetables. Vitamins are necessary for good health and can be antioxidants. Eating a balanced diet will supply all the necessary vitamins. Elderly people and people suffering from chronic diseases may not eat balanced diets and may need to supplement with vitamins. These people may not be able to absorb enough vitamins from a healthy diet. This is especially true for vitamin B3, nicotinamide, where as many as 30% of elderly people can be deficient in this vitamin.

CONCLUSIONS

Hydrogen peroxide triggers intracellular signals that activate glutathione, glutathione peroxidase, and other antioxidant response elements. This first line of defense is effective at re-establishing the balance needed for health, except in disease and patients living unhealthy lifestyles. Patients must be educated that exercise and healthy diets can quickly help re-establish good health by balancing the body's antioxidant system.

REFERENCES

[1]   Speijer D, Manjeri GR, Szklarczyk R. How to deal with oxygen radicals stemming from mitochondrial fatty acid oxidation. Philos Trans R Soc Lond B Biol Sci 2014; 369(1646): 20130446.
        [http://dx.doi.org/10.1098/rstb.2013.0446] [PMID: 24864314]

[2]   Mukherjee SK, Adams JD Jr. The effects of aging and neurodegeneration on apoptosis-associated DNA fragmentation and the benefits of nicotinamide. Mol Chem Neuropathol 1997; 32(1-3): 59-74.
        [http://dx.doi.org/10.1007/BF02815167] [PMID: 9437658]

[3]   Klaidman LK, Mukherjee SK, Adams JD Jr. Oxidative changes in brain pyridine nucleotides and neuroprotection using nicotinamide. Biochim Biophys Acta 2001; 1525(1-2): 136-48.
        [http://dx.doi.org/10.1016/S0304-4165(00)00181-1] [PMID: 11342263]

[4]   Adams J, Mukherjee S, Klaidman L, *et al.* Ischemic and metabolic stress induced apoptosis. Free Radicals in Brain Pathophysiology. New York: Marcel Dekker 2000; pp. 55-76.

[5]   Wu T, Wang XJ, Tian W, Jaramillo MC, Lau A, Zhang DD. Poly(ADP-ribose) polymerase-1 modulates Nrf2-dependent transcription. Free Radic Biol Med 2014; 67: 69-80.
        [http://dx.doi.org/10.1016/j.freeradbiomed.2013.10.806] [PMID: 24140708]

[6]   Ross D, Siegel D. NAD(P)H:quinone oxidoreductase 1 (NQO1, DT-diaphorase), functions and pharmacogenetics. Methods Enzymol 2004; 382: 115-44.
        [http://dx.doi.org/10.1016/S0076-6879(04)82008-1] [PMID: 15047100]

[7]   Mukherjee S, Sonee M, Adams J. A review of the regulatory role of nicotinamide on pro- and anti-apoptotic proteins in neuronal cells. Lett Drug Des Discov 2005; 2: 551-7.
        [http://dx.doi.org/10.2174/157018005774479177]

[8]   Lismont C, Revenco I, Fransen M. Peroxisomal hydrogen peroxide metabolism and signaling in health and disease. Int J Mol Sci 2019; 20(15): 3673.
        [http://dx.doi.org/10.3390/ijms20153673] [PMID: 31357514]

[9]   Chelikani P, Fita I, Loewen PC. Diversity of structures and properties among catalases. Cell Mol Life Sci 2004; 61(2): 192-208.
[http://dx.doi.org/10.1007/s00018-003-3206-5] [PMID: 14745498]

[10]   Kirkman HN, Galiano S, Gaetani GF. The function of catalase-bound NADPH. J Biol Chem 1987; 262(2): 660-6.
[http://dx.doi.org/10.1016/S0021-9258(19)75835-9] [PMID: 3805001]

[11]   Nagan N, Zoeller RA. Plasmalogens: biosynthesis and functions. Prog Lipid Res 2001; 40(3): 199-229.
[http://dx.doi.org/10.1016/S0163-7827(01)00003-0] [PMID: 11275267]

[12]   Franklin CC, Backos DS, Mohar I, White CC, Forman HJ, Kavanagh TJ. Structure, function, and post-translational regulation of the catalytic and modifier subunits of glutamate cysteine ligase. Mol Aspects Med 2009; 30(1-2): 86-98.
[http://dx.doi.org/10.1016/j.mam.2008.08.009] [PMID: 18812186]

[13]   Adams JD Jr, Lauterburg BH, Mitchell JR. Plasma glutathione and glutathione disulfide in the rat: regulation and response to oxidative stress. J Pharmacol Exp Ther 1983; 227(3): 749-54.
[PMID: 6655568]

[14]   Hanigan MH. Gamma-glutamyl transpeptidase: redox regulation and drug resistance. Adv Cancer Res 2014; 122: 103-41.
[http://dx.doi.org/10.1016/B978-0-12-420117-0.00003-7] [PMID: 24974180]

[15]   Adams JD, Johannessen JN, Bacon JP. Quantification of glutathione and glutathione disulfide in human plasma. Clin Chem 1987; 33(9): 1675-6.
[http://dx.doi.org/10.1093/clinchem/33.9.1675a] [PMID: 3621580]

[16]   Lauterburg BH, Adams JD, Mitchell JR. Hepatic glutathione homeostasis in the rat: efflux accounts for glutathione turnover. Hepatology 1984; 4(4): 586-90.
[http://dx.doi.org/10.1002/hep.1840040402] [PMID: 6745847]

[17]   Adams JD Jr, Lauterburg BH, Mitchell JR. Plasma glutathione disulfide as an index of oxidant stress in vivo: effects of carbon tetrachloride, dimethylnitrosamine, nitrofurantoin, metronidazole, doxorubicin and diquat. Res Commun Chem Pathol Pharmacol 1984; 46(3): 401-10.
[PMID: 6515129]

[18]   Morgan B, Ezeriņa D, Amoako TN, Riemer J, Seedorf M, Dick TP. Multiple glutathione disulfide removal pathways mediate cytosolic redox homeostasis. Nat Chem Biol 2013; 9(2): 119-25.
[http://dx.doi.org/10.1038/nchembio.1142] [PMID: 23242256]

[19]   Adams JD Jr, Wang B, Klaidman LK, LeBel CP, Odunze IN, Shah D. New aspects of brain oxidative stress induced by tert-butylhydroperoxide. Free Radic Biol Med 1993; 15(2): 195-202.
[http://dx.doi.org/10.1016/0891-5849(93)90059-4] [PMID: 8375692]

[20]   Adams JD Jr, Klaidman LK, Chang ML, Yang J. Brain oxidative stress--analytical chemistry and thermodynamics of glutathione and NADPH. Curr Top Med Chem 2001; 1(6): 473-82.
[http://dx.doi.org/10.2174/1568026013394778] [PMID: 11895124]

[21]   Schafer FQ, Buettner GR. Redox environment of the cell as viewed through the redox state of the glutathione disulfide/glutathione couple. Free Radic Biol Med 2001; 30(11): 1191-212.
[http://dx.doi.org/10.1016/S0891-5849(01)00480-4] [PMID: 11368918]

[22]   Mukherjee SK, Yasharel R, Klaidman LK, Hutchin TP, Adams JD Jr. Apoptosis and DNA fragmentation as induced by tertiary butylhydroperoxide in the brain. Brain Res Bull 1995; 38(6): 595-604.
[http://dx.doi.org/10.1016/0361-9230(96)80157-2] [PMID: 8590084]

[23]   Adams JD Jr, Klaidman LK, Huang YM, *et al.* The neuropathology of intracerebroventricular t-butylhydroperoxide. Mol Chem Neuropathol 1994; 22(2): 123-42.
[http://dx.doi.org/10.1007/BF03160100] [PMID: 7916771]

[24] Lv H, Zhen C, Liu J, Yang P, Hu L, Shang P. Unraveling the potential role of glutathione in multiple forms of cell death in cancer therapy 2019.
[http://dx.doi.org/10.1155/2019/3150145]

[25] Scirè A, Cianfruglia L, Minnelli C, *et al.* Glutathione compartmentalization and its role in glutathionylation and other regulatory processes of cellular pathways. Biofactors 2019; 45(2): 152-68.
[http://dx.doi.org/10.1002/biof.1476] [PMID: 30561781]

[26] Minich DM, Brown BI. A review of dietary (phyto)nutrients for glutathione support. Nutrients 2019; 11(9): 2073.
[http://dx.doi.org/10.3390/nu11092073] [PMID: 31484368]

[27] Elokda AS, Nielsen DH. Effects of exercise training on the glutathione antioxidant system. Eur J Cardiovasc Prev Rehabil 2007; 14(5): 630-7.
[http://dx.doi.org/10.1097/HJR.0b013e32828622d7] [PMID: 17925621]

[28] Xiong Y, Uys JD, Tew KD, Townsend DM. S-glutathionylation: from molecular mechanisms to health outcomes. Antioxid Redox Signal 2011; 15(1): 233-70.
[http://dx.doi.org/10.1089/ars.2010.3540] [PMID: 21235352]

[29] Lubos E, Loscalzo J, Handy DE. Glutathione peroxidase-1 in health and disease: from molecular mechanisms to therapeutic opportunities. Antioxid Redox Signal 2011; 15(7): 1957-97.
[http://dx.doi.org/10.1089/ars.2010.3586] [PMID: 21087145]

[30] Li C, Deng X, Xie X, Liu Y, Friedmann Angeli JP, Lai L. Activation of glutathione peroxidase 4 as a novel anti-inflammatory strategy. Front Pharmacol 2018; 9: 1120.
[http://dx.doi.org/10.3389/fphar.2018.01120] [PMID: 30337875]

[31] Su L, Zhang J, Gomez H, *et al.* Reactive oxygen species-induced lipid peroxidation in apoptosis, autophagy, and ferroptosis 2019.
[http://dx.doi.org/10.1155/2019/5080843]

[32] Begas P, Liedgens L, Moseler A, Meyer AJ, Deponte M. Glutaredoxin catalysis requires two distinct glutathione interaction sites. Nat Commun 2017; 8: 14835.
[http://dx.doi.org/10.1038/ncomms14835] [PMID: 28374771]

[33] Forman HJ, Davies MJ, Krämer AC, *et al.* Protein cysteine oxidation in redox signaling: Caveats on sulfenic acid detection and quantification. Arch Biochem Biophys 2017; 617: 26-37.
[http://dx.doi.org/10.1016/j.abb.2016.09.013] [PMID: 27693037]

[34] Perkins A, Nelson KJ, Parsonage D, Poole LB, Karplus PA. Peroxiredoxins: guardians against oxidative stress and modulators of peroxide signaling. Trends Biochem Sci 2015; 40(8): 435-45.
[http://dx.doi.org/10.1016/j.tibs.2015.05.001] [PMID: 26067716]

[35] Ince V, Carr BI, Bag HG, *et al.* Gamma glutamyl transpeptidase as a prognostic biomarker in hepatocellular cancer patients especially with >5 cm tumors, treated by liver transplantation. Int J Biol Markers 2020; 35(2): 91-5.
[http://dx.doi.org/10.1177/1724600820921869] [PMID: 32436751]

[36] Koenig G, Seneff S, van der Pol A, *et al.* 2017.

[37] Yu YM, Ryan CM, Fei ZW, *et al.* Plasma L-5-oxoproline kinetics and whole blood glutathione synthesis rates in severely burned adult humans. Am J Physiol Endocrinol Metab 2002; 282(2): E247-58.
[http://dx.doi.org/10.1152/ajpendo.00206.2001] [PMID: 11788355]

[38] Morrow JD, Hill KE, Burk RF, Nammour TM, Badr KF, Roberts LJ II. A series of prostaglandin F2-like compounds are produced in vivo in humans by a non-cyclooxygenase, free radical-catalyzed mechanism. Proc Natl Acad Sci USA 1990; 87(23): 9383-7.
[http://dx.doi.org/10.1073/pnas.87.23.9383] [PMID: 2123555]

[39] Evans AR, Junger H, Southall MD, *et al.* Isoprostanes, novel eicosanoids that produce nociception and

sensitize rat sensory neurons. J Pharmacol Exp Ther 2000; 293(3): 912-20.
[PMID: 10869392]

[40]   Davì G, Falco A, Patrono C. Determinants of F2-isoprostane biosynthesis and inhibition in man. Chem Phys Lipids 2004; 128(1-2): 149-63.
[http://dx.doi.org/10.1016/j.chemphyslip.2003.10.001] [PMID: 15037160]

[41]   Seet RC, Lee CY, Loke WM, *et al.* Biomarkers of oxidative damage in cigarette smokers: which biomarkers might reflect acute versus chronic oxidative stress? Free Radic Biol Med 2011; 50(12): 1787-93.
[http://dx.doi.org/10.1016/j.freeradbiomed.2011.03.019] [PMID: 21420490]

[42]   Elsheikh MS, Mohamed NH, Alsharkawy AAA. Improvement of asthma control after laser acupuncture and its impact on exhaled 8-isoprostane as an oxidative biomarker in chronic bronchial asthma. Respir Med 2019; 156: 15-9.
[http://dx.doi.org/10.1016/j.rmed.2019.07.022] [PMID: 31382164]

[43]   Ames PRJ, Merashli M, Bucci T, Nourooz-Zadeh J. Isoprostane in systemic sclerosis: A systematic review and meta-analysis. Mod Rheumatol 2019; 29(3): 470-5.
[http://dx.doi.org/10.1080/14397595.2018.1469458] [PMID: 29693466]

[44]   Sabanayagam C, Lye WK, Januszewski A, *et al.* Urinary isoprostane levels and age-related macular degeneration. Invest Ophthalmol Vis Sci 2017; 58(5): 2538-43.
[http://dx.doi.org/10.1167/iovs.16-21263] [PMID: 28492872]

[45]   Nikolaidis MG, Kyparos A, Vrabas IS. F_2-isoprostane formation, measurement and interpretation: the role of exercise. Prog Lipid Res 2011; 50(1): 89-103.
[http://dx.doi.org/10.1016/j.plipres.2010.10.002] [PMID: 20951733]

[46]   Patrignani P, Panara MR, Tacconelli S, *et al.* Effects of vitamin E supplementation on F(2)-isoprostane and thromboxane biosynthesis in healthy cigarette smokers. Circulation 2000; 102(5): 539-45.
[http://dx.doi.org/10.1161/01.CIR.102.5.539] [PMID: 10920066]

[47]   Roberts LJ II, Oates JA, Linton MF, *et al.* The relationship between dose of vitamin E and suppression of oxidative stress in humans. Free Radic Biol Med 2007; 43(10): 1388-93.
[http://dx.doi.org/10.1016/j.freeradbiomed.2007.06.019] [PMID: 17936185]

[48]   Sutherland WH, Manning PJ, Walker RJ, de Jong SA, Ryalls AR, Berry EA. Vitamin E supplementation and plasma 8-isoprostane and adiponectin in overweight subjects. Obesity (Silver Spring) 2007; 15(2): 386-91.
[http://dx.doi.org/10.1038/oby.2007.546] [PMID: 17299112]

[49]   Kushi LH. Vitamin E and heart disease: a case study. Am J Clin Nutr 1999; 69(6) (Suppl.): 1322S-9S.
[http://dx.doi.org/10.1093/ajcn/69.6.1322S] [PMID: 10359233]

CHAPTER 7

The Energy Balance of the Body

Abstract: The body depends on NAD to indicate/sense the energy levels in the body. When energy is normal, sirtuins respond to fluctuations in energy demands and regulate gene transcription. When the body is under an oxidative challenge, poly(ADP-ribose) polymerase responds to DNA strand breaks and increases the activities of DNA repair enzymes. NAD and ATP are closely linked in the cell since they are both high-energy adenine nucleotides and are mutually required for their own synthesis.

Keywords: Exercise, Poly(ADP-ribose) Polymerase, NAD, NADPH Oxidase, NADH Oxidase, Nicotinamide, Sirtuin.

1. INTRODUCTION

There is an energy balance in the body that depends on ATP, cAMP, NADPH, NADP, NADH and other factors. These factors protect DNA, mitochondria, proteins and lipids that are vital for cell repair and survival. They are also involved in respiration and the transportation of nutrients into cells.

NAD is an abundant molecule that exists in cells in concentrations of about 0.1 to 0.6 μmole/g of tissue [1]. It is a dinucleotide of nicotinamide and adenine linked by two high energy phosphate bonds. The beta anomer of NAD is the natural form and contains D-ribose sugars. NAD is the switch that senses energy deficits or excesses and adjusts enzyme activities and genetic expression of enzymes to reestablish energy balance [2, 3]. Two enzymes are critical to this switching process, poly(ADP-ribose) polymerase and sirtuins.

It should be mentioned that quantitating NADPH and NADH requires the proper methodology [1]. These compounds oxidize readily in biological extracts due to the presence of iron. The addition of cyanide during extraction allows cyanide to chelate iron, preventing oxidation. Cyanide also derivatizes NAD and NADP, making them fluorescent for better HPLC detection.

2. SIRTUINS

Sirtuins are the energy switches in normal cellular physiology. They respond to NAD changes and alter the activities of histones and other proteins. Sirtuins deacetylate the lysines of various enzymes, which alters their activities [4]. The mechanism of this deacetylation is shown in Fig. (**1**). However, sirtuins can also function as ADP-ribosyl transferases, which will be discussed later. Sirtuins contain a Rossman fold, a zinc-binding site and a NAD binding site [4]. The NAD binding of sirtuins leads to ADP-ribose binding to enzymes that cause lysine deacetylation and the formation of 2-O-acetyl ADP ribose (Fig. **1**). In a mechanism similar to deacetylation, sirtuins can deacylate enzymes by removing malonate, succinate, glutarate and other compounds. There are 7 human sirtuins, each with different activities and subcellular locations [5, 6] as shown in Table **1** . Each of these enzymes can be inhibited by nicotinamide, a product of enzymatic action, in a feedback mechanism. This feedback mechanism involves the fact that the enzymes can function in reverse and use nicotinamide to make NAD [4].

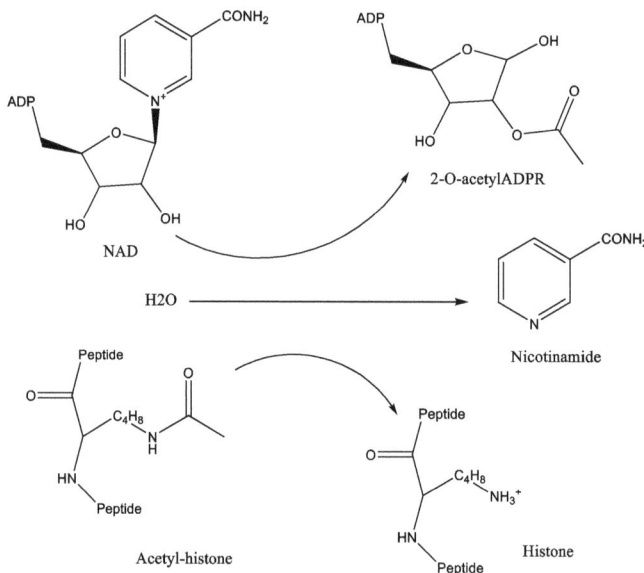

Fig. (1). Mechanism of deacetylation by sirtuins.

It should be mentioned that there are many histone deacetylase enzymes, not just sirtuins. These enzymes regulate epigenetic processes. Sirtuins bind NAD, which makes them different from other histone deacetylases. Several anticancer drugs are available that inhibit histone deacetylases: vorinostat, Panobinostat, belinostat and chidamide.

Table 1. Sirtuin subcellular locations, activities and targets. Hif is hypoxia inducible factor. MYC is a family of regulatory genes and proto-oncogenes. FOXO are the forkhead family of transcription factors. EIF are the eukaryotic initiation factors. P53 is a tumor suppressor protein. G6PD is glucose-6-phosphate dehydrogenase. SOD is superoxide dismutase. PDMC is pyruvate dehydrogenase multienzyme complex. IDH is isocitrate dehydrogenase. GOT is the gene that encodes aspartate aminotransferase. GDH is glutamate dehydrogenase. PDH is pyruvate dehydrogenase. CPS is carbamoyl phosphate synthetase. GSK is glycogen synthase kinase. LEF is lymphoid enhancer factor. PPAR-α is peroxisome proliferator activated receptor. DGAT1 is diglyceride acyltransferase. UPR is unfolded protein response. NRF is nuclear respiratory factor.

	Subcellular Location	Enzymatic Activity	Histone Target	Nonhistone Target
Sirtuin-1	Nucleus, cytoplasm	Deacetylation	H3K9Ac, H1K26Ac H4K16Ac	Hif1α, Hif2α, MYC, P53, FOXO
Sirtuin-2	Nucleus, cytoplasm	Deacetylation	H3K56Ac, H4K16Ac	Tubulin, FOXO3a, EIF5A, P53, G6PD, MYC, GSK3β
Sirtuin-3	Mitochondria	Deacetylation	H3K56Ac, H4K14Ac	SOD2, PDMC1a, IDH2, GOT2, FOXO3a
Sirtuin-4	Mitochondria	ADP-ribosylation	Unknown	GDH, PDH
Sirtuin-5	Mitochondria	Malonyl, Succinyl, Glutaryl deacylation	Unknown	CPS1
Sirtuin-6	Nucleus	Deacetylation, ADP-ribosylation, long chain fatty acid deacylation	H3K9Ac, H3K56 Ac	LEF1, PPAR-α, DGAT1
Sirtuin-7	Nucleus	Deacetylation	H3K18Ac	Hif1α, Hif2α, UPR, NRF

3. OBESITY

Sirtuins affect the activities of many genes. For instance, obesity alters the expressions of SIRT1, SIRT2, SIRT3 and SIRT6 [7]. This alters the expressions of their target genes, PPAR-α, progastricsin PGC1-α, NRF1, DGAT1, PPAR-γ and FOXO3a. This shifts the physiology of obese patients to an inflammatory status.

Decreased sirtuin-1 activity in obesity increases the activities of PPAR-γ, PGC1-α and FOXO3a. Both PPAR-α and PPAR-γ have anti-inflammatory activities [8], indicating that their upregulation is a compensatory mechanism against other inflammatory activities. PGC1-α is inflammatory in the stomach and small intestine [9] and also increases the number of mitochondria in cells [7]. Mitochondria produce reactive oxygen species that can damage cells, as will be discussed later. FOXO3a promotes and maintains inflammatory leukocyte survival [10] and can activate caspase leading to apoptosis of other cells [7]. Hif activity is decreased by the loss of sirtuin-1 activity [11]. This decreases cell repair, cell differentiation, endothelial cell growth, chondrocyte survival and many other activities.

Obesity increases sirtuin-2 activity in subdermal fat [7]. Tubulins are substrates for sirtuin-2, which may lead to changes in cellular transport processes and decreased cellular energy supplies. Increased sirtuin-2 inhibits P53 pathways and oxidative stress [12]. This is considered a salvage mechanism for cells that are severely stressed. GPDH is the primary source of NADPH in cells, which is required for the maintenance of GSH levels. Sirtuin-2 acetylates and activates GPDH [13]. Increased GPDH activity shunts the cellular metabolism of glucose into the pentose phosphate pathway. This may decrease NAD levels in order to produce more NADPH.

Sirtuin-3 decreases obesity, leading to increases in NRF1 and PCG1-α activities [7]. NRF1 regulates the expression of genes involved in cell growth, respiration, heme synthesis and mitochondrial DNA synthesis. NRF1 overexpression increases inflammatory adipokine production and insulin resistance [14]. This increases the inflammation associated with obesity.

Sirtuin-6 decreases obesity and decreases DGAT1 activity [7]. This enzyme is found mostly in enterocytes, where it makes triglycerides. Decreased triglyceride synthesis in enterocytes probably increases diglyceride levels in the blood. Diglycerides have many functions, including protein kinase C activation, transient receptor potential canonical cation channel (TRPC) activation, and precursor for prostaglandins and endocannabinoids. Endocannabinoids stimulate inflammatory adipokine production, as will be discussed later. TRPC activation causes inflammation, as will be discussed later.

4. OXIDATIVE STRESS

Sirtuins are important in maintaining homeostasis during oxidative stress as induced by reactive oxygen species [15]. The antioxidant response element (ARE) is a short sequence of DNA within a promoter region that binds transcription factors and regulates gene transcription. The ARE responds to changes in the cellular redox state and triggers responses, especially through nuclear factor E2 related factor 2 (NRF2). This, in turn, regulates several genes involved in response to oxidative stress [15].

Sirtuin-1 increases the expression of NRF2, heme oxygenase-1, and superoxide dismutase-1 [15]. Sirtuin-1 also increases P53 activity, which increases superoxide   dismutase-2 and   glutathione peroxidase-1. However, sirtuin-1

increases PGC1-α, which increases the replication of mitochondria and increases reactive oxygen species production. Hydrogen peroxide downregulates sirtuin-1.

Sirtuin-2 deacetylates NRF2 and decreases its activity [15], thereby decreasing the activity of AKT (protein kinase B). This decreases the activity of glutamate-cysteine ligase and results in decreased levels of glutathione (GSH) in the nucleus and cytoplasm. Sirtuin-2 also activates NFkB, which has several opposing effects on oxidative stress. It increases the activities of NADPH oxidase and xanthine oxidoreductase. Conversely, it increases superoxide dismutase-1 and 2, and thioredoxin activities [15].

Sirtuin-3 deacetylates several proteins involved in oxidative phosphorylation in mitochondria [16]. This appears to decrease reactive oxygen species production by mitochondria. Sirtuin-3 also increases the activities of superoxide dismutase-2 and catalase, which are protective against oxidative stress [15].

Sirtuin-4 increases reactive oxygen species generation by mitochondria [15]. Sirtuin-5 desuccinylates superoxide dismutase-1 and deacetylates cytochrome c, thereby increasing their activities [15]. This appears to decrease reactive oxygen species production. Sirtuin-6 coactivates NRF2 and activates the AMPK-FOXO3a axis [15]. This should be protective against oxidative stress.

DNA is quickly damaged by reactive oxygen species [17]. Sirtuin-1 is involved in DNA repair by nucleotide excision repair [15]. Sirtuin-1 inhibition accelerates telomere shortening. This is important in the senescence of yeast and perhaps other simple organisms. There is no evidence that this mechanism is important in human senescence.

5. EXERCISE

Physical activity is a potent activator of sirtuins [2]. Daily physical activity increases reactive oxygen species production but also induces enzymes that protect against oxidative stress, including sirtuins. Nicotinamide phosphoribosyltransferase (NAMPT) activity increases in skeletal muscle due to exercise [2]. This enzyme converts nicotinamide into nicotinamide mononucleotide (NMN) and is the rate-limiting reaction in NAD synthesis.

6. DIABETES

Sirtuin-1 expression decreases in skeletal muscle during diabetes and may be involved in insulin resistance and insulin receptor signaling [18]. The loss of sirtuin-1 activity decreases fatty acid oxidation in skeletal muscle. The accumulation of fat in the muscle causes insulin resistance. Adiponectin decreases obesity onset type 2 diabetes and is needed for sirtuin-1 activation.

Sirtuin-2 downregulation in diabetes decreases GPDH activity [18] which will decrease NADPH production, which is needed for GSH maintenance. Sirtuin-3 decreases in human pancreas cells in type 2 diabetes [18]. This may decrease the protection of mitochondria by the enzyme. There is evidence that sirtuin-6 is involved in insulin secretion and insulin sensitivity in animal models.

7. STEM CELLS

There has been considerable interest in the involvement of sirtuin activity in the growth and maintenance of stem cells. Several signaling pathways are involved in stem cell self-renewal, including a hedgehog, Wnt, and NOTCH. All of these pathways are regulated by sirtuins [2].

8. SIRTUIN INHIBITORS AND ACTIVATORS

Clearly, sirtuins are important energy switches in the body. They can also switch the body into an inflammatory status, such as in obesity and protect against reactive oxygen species. Several inhibitors and activators of sirtuins have been tested in laboratory experiments and clinical trials. There have been many publications about resveratrol, an allosteric activator of sirtuin-1, which increases lifespan in yeast and obese mice [2, 5, 19 - 21]. The obese mice were fed resveratrol at 5 or 20 mg/kg/day for 6 months [22]. This corresponds to 400 mg or 1.6 g per day in an 80 kg person. Resveratrol is a naturally occurring phenol found in some berries, nuts and other sources. It has poor bioavailability [23]. Clinical trials of resveratrol have been completed in obese patients where it increased sirtuin-1 activity, improved muscle respiration and decreased inflammation [21]. However, in men over 60 years old, resveratrol decreased the cardioprotective effects of 8 weeks of exercise and did not increase sirtuin-1 activity [21]. Similarly, post-menopausal women resveratrol did not improve metabolic parameters or increase sirtuin-1 activity [21]. Clearly, the effects of resveratrol in humans are not as favorable as in other organisms.

Metformin is a drug used in the treatment of type 2 diabetes. It inhibits mitochondrial respiratory chain complex 1, activates AMP activated protein kinase, inhibits the effects of glucagon on cAMP and protein kinase A, inhibits mitochondrial glycerophosphate dehydrogenase and has an effect on gut microbiota. Metformin also activates sirtuin-1 and decreases kidney pathology in diabetic patients [24].

Curcumin stimulates sirtuin-1 activity and has shown cardioprotective effects in a number of experimental models [21]. It extends lifespan in mice [2]. Curcumin has been used as a spice for centuries in India and other areas to extend human lifespan. Its bioavailability can be increased by black pepper. Several nanocarriers are being tested to increase the bioavailability of curcumin and other polyphenols. There are several other natural compounds that increase sirtuin-1 activity in animal models, such as berberine, quercetin, and epigallocatechin-3-gallate [21]. Cyanidin was shown to be a powerful activator of sirtuin-6 in cell preparations [20]. The bioavailability of this charged anthocyanidin is not known.

9. POLY(ADP-RIBOSE) POLYMERASE

DNA is under constant use for RNA transcription to make new proteins. Each cell makes new proteins every day to replace damaged or inactive proteins. DNA is also damaged by reactive oxygen species, especially peroxides and must be repaired [7, 25]. In fact, DNA is one of the first targets of reactive oxygen species during oxidative stress events, such as ischemia-reperfusion [7, 25].

Poly(ADP-ribose) polymerase is a switch that enables DNA repair [28, 29]. The enzyme cleaves NAD and attaches polymers of ADP-ribose to histones and other DNA repair enzymes. These polymers are positively charged, which helps DNA repair enzymes attach to negatively charged DNA. DNA damage can cause so much ADP-ribose polymerization that NAD becomes depleted [7, 25], which causes ATP depletion. Both ATP and NAD are high-energy adenine-containing compounds and depend on each other for synthesis. ATP can be made in mitochondria due to the NADH-dependent electron transport chain. NAD is made by enzymes that require ATP (Fig. **2**) . When ATP is depleted, cell death occurs either by necrosis or apoptosis [28, 29]. A small but critical amount of DNA damage causes apoptosis. More DNA damage causes necrosis.

NAD biosynthetic pathways (Fig. **2**) have been discussed and described extensively in the literature [30 - 33]. The original work by Preiss and Handler examined the conversion of nicotinamide into NAD [34]. In later work, they examined NAD synthesis from nicotinic acid, which is a minor pathway [35]. The conversion of nicotinic acid into NAD clearly starts with the conversion of nicotinic acid into nicotinamide by nicotinamidase (6), which has a Km for nicotinamide of 0.1 M [36]. Rowen and Kornberg worked earlier than Preiss and Handler and described the synthesis of nicotinamide mononucleotide from nicotinamide riboside by nicotinamide riboside kinase (2) and the phosphorolysis of nicotinamide mononucleotide by the enzyme [37]. Preiss and Handler doubted the existence of nicotinamide riboside kinase. However, there is no doubt that nicotinamide riboside is enzymatically or hydrolytically cleaved to produce nicotinamide [38] by purine nucleoside phosphorylase. More recently, it was shown that nicotinamide riboside kinase catalyzes the conversion of nicotinamide riboside into nicotinamide mononucleotide [39, 40], which confirms the earlier observation by Rowen and Kornberg.

Nicotinic acid adenine dinucleotide phosphate (NAADP) is an important calcium releasing agent since it activates voltage-sensitive two-pore channels [41]. It is made from NAD [42] and releases calcium from endolysosomes. This is very important to endothelial cell growth and function. In addition, NAADP is involved in calcium release in the heart [43]. The synthesis of NAADP in cells is regulated by histamine [40]. Other calcium-releasing agents made from NAD are cyclic ADP-ribose and adenosine diphosphoribose [42].

10. LONGEVITY

A correlation between lifespan and maximal poly(ADP-ribose) polymerase activity has been reported in several mammalian species [44]. In addition, poly(ADP-ribose) polymerase activity is 1.6 fold higher in human centenarians than younger controls [45]. This implies that the ability to repair DNA results in longer lifespan.

NAD levels decrease with aging in part because of age-associated loss of nicotinamide phosphoribosyltransferase activity (Fig. **2**) and increased NAD degradation, especially by NAD^+ nucleosidase and cyclic ADP ribose hydrolase [46]. This enzyme cleaves NAD and NADP. Aging also increases mitochondrial production of reactive oxygen species, which results in nuclear DNA damage. Protein damage increases because superoxide radical anion attacks protein thiols and converts them to thiyl radicals [47], which alters the activities of many enzymes. This will be discussed in the glutathione chapter.

The increase in poly(ADP-ribose) polymerase activity with age suggests that inhibitors of the enzyme may increase longevity. It is also possible that DNA repair is the critical event, such that increased poly(ADP-ribose) polymerase activity will increase longevity. The decrease in NAD levels with aging suggests that agents that increase NAD levels may increase longevity. So far, no inhibitor of poly(ADP-ribose) polymerase has been shown to increase longevity in humans.

About 30% of adults over the age of 70 have inadequate vitamin B_3 intake [36], which may decrease tissue NAD levels. Vitamin B_3 is both nicotinamide and nicotinic acid (niacin). Both are recognized as B vitamins even though they are pharmacologically very different. Both compounds increase tissue levels of NAD and are beneficial against pellagra-induced neurodegeneration and death [36].

11. NIACIN

Niacin is used clinically to decrease blood triglycerides and increase blood high-density lipoprotein. Niacin is not taken up in the brain. Niacin side effects include facial flushing, liver and muscle toxicity, gastrointestinal discomfort, pruritis, macular edema, stroke, ulcers, and other problems [36, 48]. It is used in doses up to 3 g per day. Niacin is a precursor for NAD but does not inhibit poly(ADP-ribose) polymerase [36, 49]. Niacin causes type 2 diabetes [50] and does not decrease mortality from cardiovascular disease [51]. Niacin dietary intake has been shown to be inversely related to the incidence of Alzheimer's disease and Parkinson's disease, perhaps due to the importance of high-density lipoprotein and vascular health in these diseases [52].

12. NICOTINAMIDE

Nicotinamide has no activity against blood triglycerides or lipoproteins. Nicotinamide does not cause the side effects caused by niacin, except gastrointestinal discomfort and perhaps infrequent, reversible hepatotoxicity [36, 49, 53]. Nicotinamide is actively transported into organs, including the brain and rapidly increases brain levels of NAD [17, 25 - 28]. Nicotinamide has been administered in doses up to 12 g per day [36]. It is an inhibitor of poly(ADP-ribose) polymerase and a precursor for NAD [36, 49]. Administration of 200 mg of nicotinamide to adult men increased whole blood NAD levels with maximum concentrations at 12 h [54]. Early-onset preeclampsia patients are currently being tested with nicotinamide in a clinical trial NCT02213094. There are also nicotinamide clinical trials of early-onset Parkinson's disease NCT03568968 and Friedrich's Ataxia NCT01589809. A clinical trial of nicotinamide in glaucoma is awaiting publication.

Type 2 diabetes is not caused by nicotinamide. The progression of type 1 diabetes may be decreased by nicotinamide [53]. Serum visfatin (extracellular nicotinamide phosphoribosyltransferase) is elevated in children with type 1 diabetes [55]. Visfatin is discussed in the lifestyle chapter, causes long-term insulin receptor dysfunction, and is involved in the causation of diabetes. Nicotinamide was found in a large clinical trial to delay the onset of type 1 diabetes [56]. Subsequent clinical trials found that nicotinamide did not delay the onset of type 1 diabetes [57]. It is not clear why the conflicting results were found.

There were several variables that were not controlled in the studies, such as body mass and daily exercise.

Nicotinamide protects the liver against acute alcohol toxicity in humans [58]. Administration of 1.25 g of nicotinamide to people before they each drank a bottle (750 mL) of wine restored the redox state of the liver and maintained normal liver functions. This work demonstrates that nicotinamide does not cause hepatotoxicity in most people but actually decreases hepatotoxicity.

Depression patients get relief from depression with supplements containing tryptophan, vitamin B6 and nicotinamide [59]. Tryptophan is a precursor for nicotinamide (Fig. **2**) and a precursor for intestinal serotonin. Blood serotonin can be taken up into the brain by a transporter [60] and may be involved in relieving depression.

Nicotinamide, 500 mg twice daily for 12 months, prevented nonmelanoma skin cancer and other skin lesions in 386 patients at risk of developing skin cancer [61]. There was a 20% decrease in basal cell carcinoma, 30% decrease in squamous cell carcinoma and overall a 23% decrease in nonmelanoma skin cancer.

13. OTHER NAD PRECURSORS

Nicotinamide riboside has been shown to increase tissue levels of NAD [62]. Nicotinamide riboside is currently in a clinical trial NCT04407390 to see if it helps patients infected with COVID-19. It is also in a clinical trial to see if it improves mitochondrial biogenesis in obesity NCT03951285. Several clinical trials have been completed with nicotinamide riboside [30]. The major side effect reported so far is flushing [30].

Oral administration of nicotinamide riboside (100, 300, or 1,000 mg) to 12 adults insignificantly increased NAD levels in peripheral blood mononuclear cells [63]. There was a significant increase in metabolites of nicotinamide, such as N-methyl nicotinamide, which suggests that nicotinamide riboside functions as a precursor for nicotinamide. A study of steady-state pharmacokinetics of nicotinamide riboside in humans found that it increases whole blood levels of NAD and nicotinamide riboside [64]. NAD levels increase two-fold at a steady state. Chronic administration of oral nicotinamide riboside, 500 mg twice daily for 6 weeks, to 24 adults, 65 years old has been reported [65]. Nicotinamide riboside was found to increase NAD levels in peripheral blood mononuclear cells. Another compound, nicotinic acid adenine dinucleotide, also increased. This indicates that nicotinic acid adenine dinucleotide is probably made from NAD [42] and may be able to later replenish NAD.

An examination of the safety of nicotinamide riboside in overweight patients found that 100, 300 or 1,000 mg orally daily for 8 weeks was tolerated [66]. There were no changes in lipoproteins or other indicators of health improvement. Whole blood NAD levels increased dose dependently as did nicotinamide and its metabolites. This is additional evidence that nicotinamide riboside is a delivery form for nicotinamide.

A study in 40 obese men, 40 – 70 years old, examined the effects of nicotinamide riboside, 1000 mg twice daily for 12 weeks, on insulin sensitivity [67]. There were no changes in insulin sensitivity, glucose production or disposal, resting energy expenditure, oxidation of lipids, or body composition.

Cow's milk, a dietary source of nicotinamide riboside, appears to increase the risk of developing type 1 diabetes [56]. This argues that nicotinamide riboside may cause or accelerate the onset of type 1 diabetes. It is also possible that milk contains another compound, such as galactose, that may cause oxidative stress and increase diabetes.

A study in 12 aged men examined the effects of 1000 mg of nicotinamide riboside daily for 21 days on muscle bioenergetics [68]. Aging is known to decrease muscle NAD levels [30]. Nicotinamide riboside increased muscle levels of nicotinic acid adenine dinucleotide and metabolites of nicotinamide. Whole blood levels increased of NAD, nicotinamide mononucleotide and nicotinamide metabolites. Urinary levels increased of nicotinamide riboside, nicotinic acid riboside and nicotinamide. There was downregulation of muscle genes associated with energy metabolism. There was no change in muscle strength or mitochondrial bioenergetics. However, there were decreases in the blood levels of inflammatory cytokines and adipokines including IL-2, IL-5, IL-6, and tumor necrosis factor α. This shows that nicotinamide riboside decreased the inflammatory state of the body.

Nicotinamide mononucleotide is a precursor for NAD in animal models [62]. At least in mice, it is taken up from the gut by a specific NMN transporter [69]. In the blood, it may be cleaved by extracellular NAD nucleosidase to nicotinamide riboside, which is taken into cells by equilibrative nucleoside transporters [38]. Injection of nicotinamide mononucleotide into mice results in increased brain NAD levels within 15 min [70]. This implies there is an active uptake system across the blood-brain barrier. Another possibility is that it is rapidly broken down to nicotinamide which has an uptake transporter into the brain [36]. There are several ongoing clinical trials for nicotinamide mononucleotide to study its safety, pharmacokinetics and effects on insulin sensitivity [62].

NAD or NADH have been used in clinical trials for many years especially in the treatment of Parkinson's disease [71]. NADH has been reported to have very favorable effects in the treatment of Parkinson's disease. This may be because it is broken down in the gut to nicotinamide which is taken up into the brain to make NAD. However, there may be NADH and NAD transporters that take these compounds intact into cells, as discussed later.

A more recent clinical trial examined NADH in the treatment of Alzheimer's disease [72]. Patients with probable Alzheimer's disease (N=26) were treated daily with 10 mg of NADH. There was no progression of cognitive decline after 6 months of treatment. Compared to placebo, the NADH patients performed better on mental function tests. The dose used, 10 mg, is very low compared to the doses of other NAD related compounds. This indicates that oral NADH is improving something other than brain NAD levels.

A safety study of intravenously infused NAD was completed in 8 adult men [73]. After 2 h of infusion, plasma NAD levels increased. Prior to this, the organs readily took up NAD or broke it down. Mammals have an uptake channel, connexin 43, that allows NAD to penetrate into cells [73]. There are several extracellular enzymes that break down NAD. Plasma nicotinamide, N-methyl nicotinamide and nicotinamide mononucleotide increased during infusion. Urinary levels of NAD and N-methyl nicotinamide increased during infusion.

N-Methylnicotinamide is a metabolite of nicotinamide and has significant biological activity, especially in endothelial cells [74]. It increases the production of NO and prostaglandin I2 which decrease thrombosis, decrease blood pressure and benefit arterial health. N-Methylnicotinamide also induces sirtuin-1 expression, regulates fatty acid metabolism and decreases homocysteine secretion. Inflammatory adipokines such as tumor necrosis factor α and IL-6 induce N-methyltransferase [74], which increases N-methyl nicotinamide formation, perhaps as a mechanism to inhibit further inflammation. Niacin also increases N-methyltransferase activity.

14. POLY(ADP-RIBOSE) POLYMERASE INHIBITORS

Poly(ADP-ribose) polymerase is important to the survival of cancer cells. Olaparib was approved for use against advanced ovarian cancer in 2014, metastatic breast cancer in 2018, and metastatic pancreatic cancer in 2019 [75]. A 2020 clinical trial found that Olaparib improves survival time in metastatic prostate cancer. Olaparib inhibits poly(ADP-ribose) polymerase and kills cancer cells in cancers that depend on the enzyme for DNA repair [75].

Nicotinamide has been used for many years in the cure of pellagra [36]. It increases intracellular NAD levels but is also an inhibitor of poly(ADP-ribose) polymerase. It is possible that both activities are critical to the therapy provided by nicotinamide.

15. NADPH OXIDASE

NADPH oxidases are a family of transmembrane enzymes that transfers electrons from intracellular NADPH to extracellular or intracellular oxygen, making reactive oxygen species [76]. Cytosolic NADPH is mostly generated by glucose-6-phosphate dehydrogenase, which depends on glucose as a precursor. When blood glucose levels are high, such as in diabetes, NADPH oxidases become active and can damage endothelial cells and other cells, leading to diabetic retinopathy [76], heart failure [77], Alzheimer's disease [78, 79] and stroke [80]. Damage to endothelial cells makes arteries leaky and interferes with oxygen and nutrient use. A number of NADPH oxidase inhibitors are being tested in clinical trials [76, 79]. Cilostazol is an NADPH inhibitor used in some countries to prevent stroke [78]. Clinical trials with cilostazol have shown some efficacy in early Alzheimer's disease [78]. Cilostazol is a phosphodiesterase inhibitor and has other activities as well. Apocynin is a natural compound isolated from *Apocynum cannabinum*, is an NADPH inhibitor and is active against animal models of diabetic retinopathy [76].

16. NADH OXIDASE

NAM 1→ NMN 2→ NAD 3→ NADH 4→ NAD + Superoxide Radical Anion

NADH oxidase is an extracellular enzyme bound to endothelial cells that generate reactive oxygen species in the plasma from extracellular NADH [81, 82]. NADH is made in the blood through the actions of visfatin, ecto-5'-nucleotidase and xanthine dehydrogenase [82]. Blood levels of visfatin are high in Alzheimer's disease, as are blood levels of ceramide [81]. Ceramide induces NADPH oxidase activity [81]. Visfatin (1) activity in the blood and extracellular compartments has been shown in several publications to make extracellular nicotinamide mononucleotide [33, 83, 84]. Ecto-5'-nucleotidase (2) is known to convert various mononucleotides into dinucleotides, such as NAD, and is found on the extracellular surfaces of endothelial and other cells [85]. NAD can be released from and taken up by some cells, such as muscle cells [86]. In fact, with aging extracellular NADH levels increase [87]. Xanthine dehydrogenase (3) makes NADH. NADH oxidase (4) oxidizes NADH and makes a superoxide radical anion, which dismutases to form hydrogen peroxide. Hydrogen peroxide is permeable to cell membranes and rapidly damages nuclear DNA, as discussed previously. The combination of NADH oxidase and NADPH oxidase activities generates reactive oxygen species that damage the blood-brain barrier accelerating brain deterioration. It is possible that Alzheimer's disease and Parkinson's disease are caused by leaky blood-brain barriers or are accelerated by leaky blood-brain barriers.

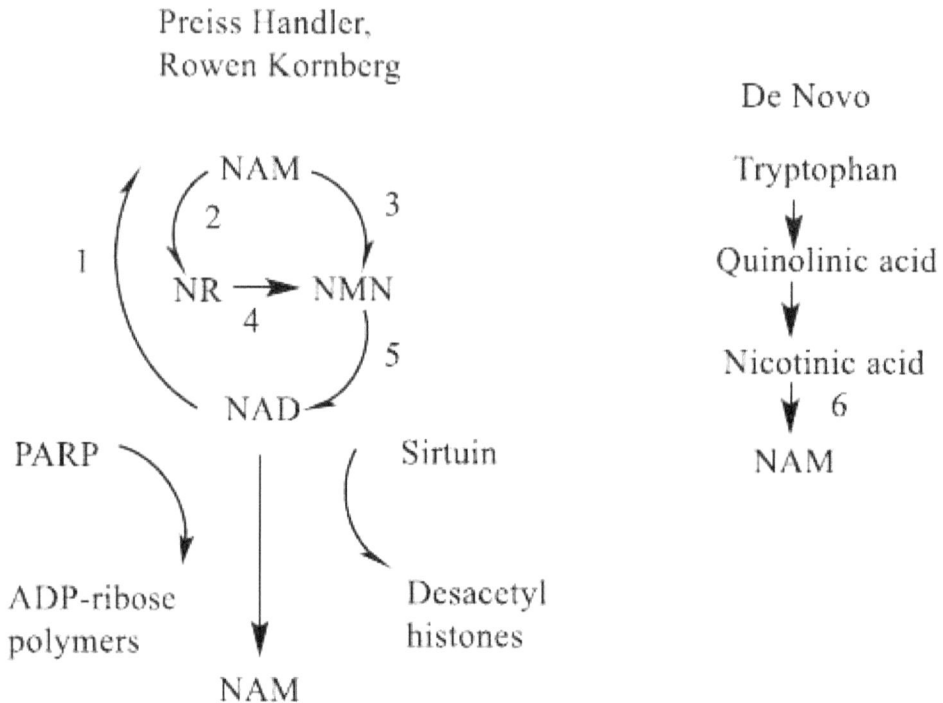

Fig. (2). NAD synthetic pathways. 1 NAD is catabolized to nicotinamide (NAM) by NAD$^+$ nucleosidase. 2 NAM is converted to nicotinamide riboside (NR) by purine nucleoside phosphorylase which requires ATP. 3 Nicotinamide is converted into nicotinamide mononucleotide (NMN) by nicotinamide phosphoribosyl transferase. It is the rate limiting enzyme in NAD synthesis. Its extracellular form is called visfatin. 4 NR is converted to NMN by nicotinamide riboside kinase which requires ATP. 5 NMN is converted to NAD by nicotinamide nucleotide adenylyltransferase which requires ATP. 6 Nicotinamidase rapidly converts nicotinic acid into nicotinamide. It does not normally function in reverse.

CONCLUSIONS

Sirtuins and poly(ADP-ribose) polymerase protect the body from damage by reactive oxygen species. Nicotinamide and NAD are necessary for their activities. These enzymes are intracellular switches that activate or deactivate the machinery needed to repair DNA and keep cellular homeostasis intact. Healthy lifestyles maximize the abilities of these switches for function.

REFERENCES

[1]   Klaidman LK, Leung AC, Adams JD Jr. High-performance liquid chromatography analysis of oxidized and reduced pyridine dinucleotides in specific brain regions. Anal Biochem 1995; 228(2): 312-7.
      [http://dx.doi.org/10.1006/abio.1995.1356] [PMID: 8572312]

[2]   Grabowska W, Sikora E, Bielak-Zmijewska A. Sirtuins, a promising target in slowing down the ageing process. Biogerontology 2017; 18(4): 447-76.
      [http://dx.doi.org/10.1007/s10522-017-9685-9] [PMID: 28258519]

[3]   Yang J, Adams J. Structure activity relationships for nicotinamide in the treatment of stroke. Lett Drug Des Discov 2004; 1: 58-65.
      [http://dx.doi.org/10.2174/1570180043485716]

[4]   Sauve AA. Sirtuin chemical mechanisms. Biochim Biophys Acta 2010; 1804(8): 1591-603.
      [http://dx.doi.org/10.1016/j.bbapap.2010.01.021] [PMID: 20132909]

[5]   Carafa V, Rotili D, Forgione M, *et al.* Sirtuin functions and modulation: from chemistry to the clinic. Clin Epigenetics 2016; 8: 61-82.
      [http://dx.doi.org/10.1186/s13148-016-0224-3] [PMID: 27226812]

[6]   O'Callaghan C, Vassilopoulos A. Sirtuins at the crossroads of stemness, aging, and cancer. Aging Cell 2017; 16(6): 1208-18.
      [http://dx.doi.org/10.1111/acel.12685] [PMID: 28994177]

[7]   Martínez-Jiménez V, Cortez-Espinosa N, Rodríguez-Varela E, *et al.* Altered levels of sirtuin genes (SIRT1, SIRT2, SIRT3 and SIRT6) and their target genes in adipose tissue from individual with obesity. Diabetes Metab Syndr 2019; 13(1): 582-9.
      [http://dx.doi.org/10.1016/j.dsx.2018.11.011] [PMID: 30641770]

[8]   Wahli W, Michalik L. PPARs at the crossroads of lipid signaling and inflammation. Trends Endocrinol Metab 2012; 23(7): 351-63.
      [http://dx.doi.org/10.1016/j.tem.2012.05.001] [PMID: 22704720]

[9]   Axelsson CK. Clinical implications of serum pepsinogen and progastricsin in man. Scand J Clin Lab Invest Suppl 1992; 210 (Suppl. 210): 81-96.
      [http://dx.doi.org/10.1080/00365519209104657] [PMID: 1455183]

[10] Peng SL. Forkhead transcription factors in chronic inflammation. Int J Biochem Cell Biol 2010; 42(4): 482-5.
      [http://dx.doi.org/10.1016/j.biocel.2009.10.013] [PMID: 19850149]

[11] Dioum EM, Chen R, Alexander MS, *et al.* Regulation of hypoxia-inducible factor 2alpha signaling by the stress-responsive deacetylase sirtuin 1. Science 2009; 324(5932): 1289-93.
      [http://dx.doi.org/10.1126/science.1169956] [PMID: 19498162]

[12] Yang M, Peng Y, Liu W, *et al.* Sirtuin 2 expression suppresses oxidative stress and senescence of nucleus pulposus cells through inhibition of the p53/p21 pathway. Biochem Biophys Res Commun 2019; 513(3): 616-22.
      [http://dx.doi.org/10.1016/j.bbrc.2019.03.200] [PMID: 30981502]

[13] Wu LE, Sinclair DA. SIRT2 controls the pentose phosphate switch. EMBO J 2014; 33(12): 1287-8.
      [http://dx.doi.org/10.15252/embj.201488713] [PMID: 24825350]

[14] van Tienen FH, Lindsey PJ, van der Kallen CJ, Smeets HJ. Prolonged Nrf1 overexpression triggers adipocyte inflammation and insulin resistance. J Cell Biochem 2010; 111(6): 1575-85.
      [http://dx.doi.org/10.1002/jcb.22889] [PMID: 21053274]

[15] Singh CK, Chhabra G, Ndiaye MA, Garcia-Peterson LM, Mack NJ, Ahmad N. The Role of Sirtuins in Antioxidant and Redox Signaling. Antioxid Redox Signal 2018; 28(8): 643-61.
      [http://dx.doi.org/10.1089/ars.2017.7290] [PMID: 28891317]

[16] Finley LW, Haigis MC. Metabolic regulation by SIRT3: implications for tumorigenesis. Trends Mol Med 2012; 18(9): 516-23.
      [http://dx.doi.org/10.1016/j.molmed.2012.05.004] [PMID: 22749020]

[17] Mukherjee SK, Klaidman LK, Yasharel R, Adams JD Jr. Increased brain NAD prevents neuronal apoptosis in vivo. Eur J Pharmacol 1997; 330(1): 27-34.
      [http://dx.doi.org/10.1016/S0014-2999(97)00171-4] [PMID: 9228411]

[18] Kitada M, Ogura Y, Monno I, Koya D. Sirtuins and type 2 diabetes: role in inflammation, oxidative stress and mitochondrial function. Front Endocrinol (Lausanne) 2019; 10: 187.
      [http://dx.doi.org/10.3389/fendo.2019.00187] [PMID: 30972029]

[19] Dai H, Sinclair DA, Ellis JL, Steegborn C. Sirtuin activators and inhibitors: Promises, achievements, and challenges. Pharmacol Ther 2018; 188: 140-54.
      [http://dx.doi.org/10.1016/j.pharmthera.2018.03.004] [PMID: 29577959]

[20] Rahnasto-Rilla M, Tyni J, Huovinen M, *et al.* Natural polyphenols as sirtuin 6 modulators. Sci Rep 2018; 8(1): 4163.
      [http://dx.doi.org/10.1038/s41598-018-22388-5] [PMID: 29515203]

[21] Treviño-Saldaña N, García-Rivas G. Regulation of Sirtuin-Mediated Protein Deacetylation by Cardioprotective Phytochemicals. Oxidative Med Cellular Longevity 2017; 16.
      [http://dx.doi.org/10.1155/2017/1750306]

[22] Baur J, Pearson K, Price N, *et al.* Resveratrol improves health and survival of mice on a high-calorie diet. Nature volume 2006; 444: 337-42.
      [http://dx.doi.org/10.1038/nature05354]

[23] Adams JD, Klaidman LK. Sirtuins, nicotinamide and aging: a critical review. Lett Drug Des Discov 2007; 4: 44-8.
      [http://dx.doi.org/10.2174/157018007778992892]

[24] Bazyluk A, Malyszko J, Hryszko T, Zbroch E. State of the art - sirtuin 1 in kidney pathology - clinical relevance. Adv Med Sci 2019; 64(2): 356-64.
      [http://dx.doi.org/10.1016/j.advms.2019.04.005] [PMID: 31125865]

[25] Chang ML, Yang J, Kem S, *et al.* Nicotinamide and ketamine reduce infarct volume and DNA fragmentation in rats after brain ischemia and reperfusion. Neurosci Lett 2002; 322(3): 137-40.
      [http://dx.doi.org/10.1016/S0304-3940(01)02520-4] [PMID: 11897157]

[26] Yang J, Klaidman LK, Chang ML, *et al.* Nicotinamide therapy protects against both necrosis and apoptosis in a stroke model. Pharmacol Biochem Behav 2002; 73(4): 901-10.
      [http://dx.doi.org/10.1016/S0091-3057(02)00939-5] [PMID: 12213537]

[27] Yang J, Klaidman LK, Nalbandian A, *et al.* The effects of nicotinamide on energy metabolism following transient focal cerebral ischemia in Wistar rats. Neurosci Lett 2002; 333(2): 91-4.
      [http://dx.doi.org/10.1016/S0304-3940(02)01005-4] [PMID: 12419488]

[28] Klaidman LK, Mukherjee SK, Adams JD Jr. Oxidative changes in brain pyridine nucleotides and neuroprotection using nicotinamide. Biochim Biophys Acta 2001; 1525(1-2): 136-48.
      [http://dx.doi.org/10.1016/S0304-4165(00)00181-1] [PMID: 11342263]

[29] Adams J, Klaidman L, Morales M, *et al.* Nicotinamide and neuroprotection Chemicals and Neurodegenerative Diseases. Dubai: Prominent Press 1999; pp. 230-60.

[30] Okabe K, Yaku K, Tobe K, Nakagawa T. Implications of altered NAD metabolism in metabolic disorders. J Biomed Sci 2019; 26(1): 34.
      [http://dx.doi.org/10.1186/s12929-019-0527-8] [PMID: 31078136]

[31]   Dölle C, Skoge RH, Vanlinden MR, Ziegler M. NAD biosynthesis in humans--enzymes, metabolites and therapeutic aspects. Curr Top Med Chem 2013; 13(23): 2907-17.
[http://dx.doi.org/10.2174/15680266113136660206] [PMID: 24171775]

[32]   Rajman L, Chwalek K, Sinclair DA. Therapeutic potential of NAD-boosting molecules: The *in vivo* evidence. Cell Metab 2018; 27(3): 529-47.
[http://dx.doi.org/10.1016/j.cmet.2018.02.011] [PMID: 29514064]

[33]   Xiao W, Wang RS, Handy DE, Loscalzo J. NAD(H) and NADP(H) redox couples and cellular energy metabolism. Antioxid Redox Signal 2018; 28(3): 251-72.
[http://dx.doi.org/10.1089/ars.2017.7216] [PMID: 28648096]

[34]   Preiss J, Handler P. Enzymatic synthesis of nicotinamide mononucleotide. J Biol Chem 1957; 225(2): 759-70.
[http://dx.doi.org/10.1016/S0021-9258(18)64875-6] [PMID: 13416279]

[35]   Mori V, Amici A, Mazzola F, *et al.* Metabolic profiling of alternative NAD biosynthetic routes in mouse tissues. PLoS One 2014; 9(11): e113939.
[http://dx.doi.org/10.1371/journal.pone.0113939] [PMID: 25423279]

[36]   Yang J, Adams J. Nicotinamide and its pharmacological properties for clinical therapy. Drug Des Rev 2004; 1: 43-52.
[http://dx.doi.org/10.2174/1567269043480726]

[37]   Rowen JW, Kornberg A. The phosphorolysis of nicotinamide riboside. J Biol Chem 1951; 193(2): 497-507.
[http://dx.doi.org/10.1016/S0021-9258(18)50905-4] [PMID: 14907738]

[38]   Poddar SK, Sifat AE, Haque S, Nahid NA, Chowdhury S, Mehedi I. Nicotinamide mononucleotide: Exploration of diverse therapeutic applications of a potential molecule. Biomolecules 2019; 9(1): 34.
[http://dx.doi.org/10.3390/biom9010034] [PMID: 30669679]

[39]   Burgos ES, Schramm VL. Weak coupling of ATP hydrolysis to the chemical equilibrium of human nicotinamide phosphoribosyltransferase. Biochemistry 2008; 47(42): 11086-96.
[http://dx.doi.org/10.1021/bi801198m] [PMID: 18823127]

[40]   Ratajczak J, Joffraud M, Trammell SA, *et al.* NRK1 controls nicotinamide mononucleotide and nicotinamide riboside metabolism in mammalian cells. Nat Commun 2016; 7: 13103.
[http://dx.doi.org/10.1038/ncomms13103] [PMID: 27725675]

[41]   Moccia F, Negri S, Shekha M, Faris P, Guerra G. Endothelial Ca2+ signaling, angiogenesis and vasculogenesis: just what it takes to make a blood vessel. Int J Mol Sci 2019; 20(16): 3962.
[http://dx.doi.org/10.3390/ijms20163962] [PMID: 31416282]

[42]   Guse AH. Calcium mobilizing second messengers derived from NAD. Biochim Biophys Acta 2015; 1854(9): 1132-7.
[http://dx.doi.org/10.1016/j.bbapap.2014.12.015] [PMID: 25534250]

[43]   Terrar DA. Calcium signaling in the heart. Adv Exp Med Biol 2020; 1131: 395-443.
[http://dx.doi.org/10.1007/978-3-030-12457-1_16] [PMID: 31646519]

[44]   Grube K, Bürkle A. Poly(ADP-ribose) polymerase activity in mononuclear leukocytes of 13 mammalian species correlates with species-specific life span. Proc Natl Acad Sci USA 1992; 89(24): 11759-63.
[http://dx.doi.org/10.1073/pnas.89.24.11759] [PMID: 1465394]

[45]   Muiras ML, Müller M, Schächter F, Bürkle A. Increased poly(ADP-ribose) polymerase activity in lymphoblastoid cell lines from centenarians. J Mol Med (Berl) 1998; 76(5): 346-54.
[http://dx.doi.org/10.1007/s001090050226] [PMID: 9587069]

[46]   Bradshaw PC. Cytoplasmic and mitochondrial NADPH-coupled redox systems in the regulation of aging. Nutrients 2019; 11(3): 504-38.

[http://dx.doi.org/10.3390/nu11030504] [PMID: 30818813]

[47]   Asada K, Kanematsu S. Reactivity of thiols with superoxide radicals. Agric Biol Chem 1976; 40: 1891-2.

[48]   https://ods.od.nih.gov/factsheets/Niacin-HealthProfessional/

[49]   Yang J, Adams J. Structure activity relationships for nicotinamide in treatment of stroke. Lett Drug Des Discov 2004; 1: 58-65.
[http://dx.doi.org/10.2174/1570180043485716]

[50]   Goldie C, Taylor AJ, Nguyen P, McCoy C, Zhao XQ, Preiss D. Niacin therapy and the risk of new-onset diabetes: a meta-analysis of randomised controlled trials. Heart 2016; 102(3): 198-203.
[http://dx.doi.org/10.1136/heartjnl-2015-308055] [PMID: 26370223]

[51]   Schandelmaier S, Briel M, Saccilotto R, *et al.* Niacin for primary and secondary prevention of cardiovascular events. Cochrane Database Syst Rev 2017; 6: CD009744.
[http://dx.doi.org/10.1002/14651858.CD009744.pub2] [PMID: 28616955]

[52]   Fricker RA, Green EL, Jenkins SI, Griffin SM. The influence of nicotinamide on health and disease in the central nervous system. Int J Tryptophan Res 2018; 11: 1178646918776658.
[http://dx.doi.org/10.1177/1178646918776658] [PMID: 29844677]

[53]   Knip M, Douek IF, Moore WP, *et al.* Safety of high-dose nicotinamide: a review. Diabetologia 2000; 43(11): 1337-45.
[http://dx.doi.org/10.1007/s001250051536] [PMID: 11126400]

[54]   Ito T, Sato T, Hakamata A, *et al.* A nonrandomized study of single oral supplementation within the daily tolerable upper level of nicotinamide affects blood nicotinamide and NAD+ levels in healthy subjects. Transl Med Aging 2020; 4: 45-54.
[http://dx.doi.org/10.1016/j.tma.2020.04.002]

[55]   Kamal M, Abbasy AJ, Muslemani AA, Bener A. Effect of nicotinamide on newly diagnosed type 1 diabetic children. Acta Pharmacol Sin 2006; 27(6): 724-7.
[http://dx.doi.org/10.1111/j.1745-7254.2006.00313.x] [PMID: 16723091]

[56]   Nurten E, Vogel M, Michael Kapellen T, *et al.* Omentin-1 and NAMPT serum concentrations are higher and CK-18 levels are lower in children and adolescents with type 1 diabetes when compared to healthy age, sex and BMI matched controls. J Pediatr Endocrinol Metab 2018; 31(9): 959-69.
[http://dx.doi.org/10.1515/jpem-2018-0353] [PMID: 30179852]

[57]   Skyler JS. Primary and secondary prevention of Type 1 diabetes. Diabet Med 2013; 30(2): 161-9.
[http://dx.doi.org/10.1111/dme.12100] [PMID: 23231526]

[58]   Volpi E, Lucidi P, Cruciani G, *et al.* Nicotinamide counteracts alcohol-induced impairment of hepatic protein metabolism in humans. J Nutr 1997; 127(11): 2199-204.
[http://dx.doi.org/10.1093/jn/127.11.2199] [PMID: 9349848]

[59]   Tsujita N, Akamatsu Y, Nishida MM, Hayashi T, Moritani T. Effect of tryptophan, vitamin B 6, and nicotinamide-containing supplement loading between meals on mood and autonomic nervous system activity in young adults with subclinical depression: A randomized, double-blind, and placebo-controlled study. J Nutr Sci Vitaminol (Tokyo) 2019; 65(6): 507-14.
[http://dx.doi.org/10.3177/jnsv.65.507] [PMID: 31902864]

[60]   Lesch K, Wolozin B, Murphy D, Riederer P. Primary structure of the human platelet serotonin uptake site: Identity with the brain serotonin transporter. J Neurochem 1993; 60: 2319-22.

[61]   Chen AC, Martin AJ, Choy B, *et al.* A phase 3 randomized trial of nicotinamide for skin-cancer chemoprevention. N Engl J Med 2015; 373(17): 1618-26.
[http://dx.doi.org/10.1056/NEJMoa1506197] [PMID: 26488693]

[62]   Mehmel M, Jovanović N, Spitz U. Nicotinamide riboside-the current state of research and therapeutic uses. Nutrients 2020; 12(6): 1616.

[http://dx.doi.org/10.3390/nu12061616] [PMID: 32486488]

[63]   Trammell S, Schmidt M, Weidemann B, *et al.* Nicotinamide riboside is uniquely and orally bioavailable in mice and humans. Nature Commun 7: 12948.2016;
[http://dx.doi.org/10.1038/ncomms12948]

[64]   Airhart SE, Shireman LM, Risler LJ, *et al.* An open-label, non-randomized study of the pharmacokinetics of the nutritional supplement nicotinamide riboside (NR) and its effects on blood NAD+ levels in healthy volunteers. PLoS One 2017; 12(12): e0186459.
[http://dx.doi.org/10.1371/journal.pone.0186459] [PMID: 29211728]

[65]   Martens CR, Denman BA, Mazzo MR, *et al.* Chronic nicotinamide riboside supplementation is well-tolerated and elevates NAD$^+$ in healthy middle-aged and older adults. Nat Commun 2018; 9(1): 1286.
[http://dx.doi.org/10.1038/s41467-018-03421-7] [PMID: 29599478]

[66]   Conze D, Brenner C, Kruger CL. Safety and metabolism of longterm administration of Niagen (nicotinamide riboside chloride) in a randomized, double-blind, placebo-controlled clinical trial of healthy overweight adults. Sci Rep 2019; 9(1): 9772.
[http://dx.doi.org/10.1038/s41598-019-46120-z] [PMID: 31278280]

[67]   Dollerup OL, Christensen B, Svart M, *et al.* A randomized placebo-controlled clinical trial of nicotinamide riboside in obese men: safety, insulin-sensitivity, and lipid-mobilizing effects. Am J Clin Nutr 2018; 108(2): 343-53.
[http://dx.doi.org/10.1093/ajcn/nqy132] [PMID: 29992272]

[68]   Elhassan YS, Kluckova K, Fletcher RS, *et al.* Nicotinamide riboside augments the aged human skeletal muscle NAD+ metabolome and induces transcriptomic and anti-inflammatory signatures. Cell Rep 2019; 28(7): 1717-1728.e6.
[http://dx.doi.org/10.1016/j.celrep.2019.07.043] [PMID: 31412242]

[69]   Grozio A, Mills KF, Yoshino J, *et al.* Slc12a8 is a nicotinamide mononucleotide transporter. Nat Metab 2019; 1(1): 47-57.
[http://dx.doi.org/10.1038/s42255-018-0009-4] [PMID: 31131364]

[70]   Yoshino J, Baur JA, Imai SI. Imai S. NAD+ intermediates: The biology and therapeutic potential of NMN and NR. Cell Metab 2018; 27(3): 513-28.
[http://dx.doi.org/10.1016/j.cmet.2017.11.002] [PMID: 29249689]

[71]   Birkmayer GJ, Birkmayer W. Stimulation of endogenous L-dopa biosynthesis--a new principle for the therapy of Parkinson's disease. The clinical effect of nicotinamide adenine dinucleotide (NADH) and nicotinamide adenine dinucleotidephosphate (NADPH). Acta Neurol Scand Suppl 1989; 126: 183-7.
[http://dx.doi.org/10.1111/j.1600-0404.1989.tb01800.x] [PMID: 2618590]

[72]   Demarin V, Podobnik SS, Storga-Tomic D, Kay G. Treatment of Alzheimer's disease with stabilized oral nicotinamide adenine dinucleotide: a randomized, double-blind study. Drugs Exp Clin Res 2004; 30(1): 27-33.
[PMID: 15134388]

[73]   Grant R, Berg J, Mestayer R, *et al.* A pilot study investigating changes in the human plasma and urine NAD+ metabolome during a 6 hour intravenous infusion of NAD+. Front Aging Neurosci 2019; 11: 257.
[http://dx.doi.org/10.3389/fnagi.2019.00257] [PMID: 31572171]

[74]   Nejabati HR, Mihanfar A, Pezeshkian M, *et al.* N1-methylnicotinamide (MNAM) as a guardian of cardiovascular system. J Cell Physiol 2018; 233(10): 6386-94.
[http://dx.doi.org/10.1002/jcp.26636] [PMID: 29741779]

[75]   Fong PC, Boss DS, Yap TA, *et al.* Inhibition of poly(ADP-ribose) polymerase in tumors from BRCA mutation carriers. N Engl J Med 2009; 361(2): 123-34.
[http://dx.doi.org/10.1056/NEJMoa0900212] [PMID: 19553641]

[76]   Peng JJ, Xiong SQ, Ding LX, Peng J, Xia XB. Diabetic retinopathy: Focus on NADPH oxidase and its

potential as therapeutic target. Eur J Pharmacol 2019; 853: 381-7.
[http://dx.doi.org/10.1016/j.ejphar.2019.04.038] [PMID: 31009636]

[77]   Wang K, Zhu ZF, Chi RF, *et al.* The NADPH oxidase inhibitor apocynin improves cardiac sympathetic nerve terminal innervation and function in heart failure. Exp Physiol 2019; 104(11): 1638-49.
[http://dx.doi.org/10.1113/EP087552] [PMID: 31475749]

[78]   Ono K, Tsuji M. Pharmacological potential of cilostazol for Alzheimer's disease. Front Pharmacol 2019; 10: 559.
[http://dx.doi.org/10.3389/fphar.2019.00559] [PMID: 31191308]

[79]   Tarafdar A, Pula G. The role of NADPH oxidases and oxidative stress in neurodegenerative disorders. Int J Mol Sci 2018; 19(12): 3824.
[http://dx.doi.org/10.3390/ijms19123824] [PMID: 30513656]

[80]   Shen J, Rastogi R, Geng X, Ding Y. Nicotinamide adenine dinucleotide phosphate oxidase activation and neuronal death after ischemic stroke. Neural Regen Res 2019; 14(6): 948-53.
[http://dx.doi.org/10.4103/1673-5374.250568]

[81]   Adams J. The treatment of brain inflammation in Alzheimer's disease. Can traditional medicines help? Front Clin Drug Res Alzheimer Disorders 2016; 6: 1-19.

[82]   Adams J. DNA, nuclear cell signaling and neurodegeneration. Extracellular and Intracellular Signaling. London: Royal Society of Chemistry 2011; pp. 175-87.
[http://dx.doi.org/10.1039/9781849733434-00175]

[83]   Garten A, Schuster S, Penke M, Gorski T, de Giorgis T, Kiess W. Physiological and pathophysiological roles of NAMPT and NAD metabolism. Nat Rev Endocrinol 2015; 11(9): 535-46.
[http://dx.doi.org/10.1038/nrendo.2015.117] [PMID: 26215259]

[84]   Yano M, Akazawa H, Oka T, *et al.* Monocyte-derived extracellular Nampt-dependent biosynthesis of NAD(+) protects the heart against pressure overload. Sci Rep 2015; 5: 15857.
[http://dx.doi.org/10.1038/srep15857] [PMID: 26522369]

[85]   Grozio A, Sociali G, Sturla L, *et al.* CD73 protein as a source of extracellular precursors for sustained NAD+ biosynthesis in FK866-treated tumor cells. J Biol Chem 2013; 288(36): 25938-49.
[http://dx.doi.org/10.1074/jbc.M113.470435] [PMID: 23880765]

[86]   Goody MF, Henry CA. A need for NAD+ in muscle development, homeostasis, and aging. Skelet Muscle 2018; 8(1): 9.
[http://dx.doi.org/10.1186/s13395-018-0154-1] [PMID: 29514713]

[87]   Clement J, Wong M, Poljak A, Sachdev P, Braidy N. The plasma NAD+ metabolome Is dysregulated in "normal" aging. Rejuvenation Res 2019; 22(2): 121-30.
[http://dx.doi.org/10.1089/rej.2018.2077] [PMID: 30124109]

SUBJECT INDEX

A

Abuse 1, 35, 43, 44, 45
  children 43, 44
  neglect 44
  sexual 1, 44
Abusive language 41
Acatalasemia 83
Accelerating brain deterioration 110
Acetaldehyde induction 10
Acid(S) 10, 63, 68, 69, 83, 88, 89, 90, 91, 103, 105, 110
  acetic 10
  arachidonic 63, 88, 91
  cannabidiolic 69
  linolenic 88
  nicotinic 103, 105, 110
  protein sulfenic 89
  pyroglutamic 90
  retinoic 52
  valproic 68
Activators 56, 102, 103
  allosteric 102
Activities 10, 52, 66, 69, 71, 73, 75, 83, 89, 90, 99, 104
  anticancer 52
  anti-inflammatory 52, 99
  cancer-causing 10
  catalase 83
  cyclooxygenase-2 52, 75
  enzymatic 89, 99
  immune cell 52, 73
  inflammatory 66, 99
  inhibitory 71
  neuronal 71
  nicotinamide phosphoriboxyltransferase 104
  peroxiredoxin 89
  serum γ-glutamyl transferase 90
Adenosine diphosphoribose 104
Adhesion 7, 50, 70, 91
  leukocyte 50, 70
  molecule expression 50

neutrophil 91
Adipogenesis 50
Adipokines 7, 9
  leptin 7
  visfatin 9
Adipokine secretion 70, 73
  lower inflammatory 70
  synoviocytes stimulate 73
Adipokine synthesis 7, 73
  inflammatory 7
Adiponectin production 63
Adipotoxicity 7
ADP 98 99
  ribosylation 99
  ribosyl transferases 98
ADP-ribose 82, 83, 97, 103, 104, 105, 108, 109, 110
  cyclic 104
  polymerization 103
Adrenocorticotropic hormone 56
Age-associated thymus degeneration 55
AIDS dementia 71
Alcohol 2, 10
  consumption 2, 10
  dehydrogenase 10
Aldehyde dehydrogenase 10
Alzheimer's disease 5, 41, 54, 57, 105, 108, 109
  ameliorate 41
Angiogenesis 52
Angiotensin 8
Antidepressant drugs 42
Anti-inflammatory 49, 63, 65
  drugs 63, 65
  effect 49
Antioxidants 82, 92, 93
Antipsychotic 43
  drugs 43
  medication 43
Arthritis 1, 3, 5, 9, 11, 18, 26, 57, 61, 73
  gonorrhea-induced 26
  rheumatoid 9, 57, 73

www.ingramcontent.com/pod-product-compliance
Lightning Source LLC
Chambersburg PA
CBHW060813270326
41929CB00002B/20